Praise for *The Energy Medicine Yoga Prescription*

"What I love about Lauren Walker's work and *The Energy Medicine Yoga Prescription* is that it offers simple tools to help anyone get their energy working for them, which means no more 'rowing upstream against the current.'"

SEANE CORN
cofounder of Off the Mat, Into the World®

"Lauren Walker's *The Energy Medicine Yoga Prescription* teaches us to rebalance our subtlest energies and heal from the inside out. With this vital reference, you will learn how to cultivate an authentic connection to yourself, build stellar habits, and develop a real relationship to your own wellness."

ELENA BROWER
author of *Art of Attention* and *Practice You*

"By marrying tantra yoga and Energy Medicine, Lauren Walker has created a unique path to healing, a path of love. By using her brilliant and accessible energy techniques, we can all activate our internal 'prescriptions' for health and restore balance—body, mind, and spirit."

CYNDI DALE
author of *The Subtle Body, The Subtle Body Practice Manual,* and *The Subtle Body Coloring Book*

"Prescriptions usually involve medications to help overcome illness. Medications change the body's chemistry and electromagnetic energy flows. This wonderful book teaches you how to do that using a different kind of prescription, one that is totally natural and has no adverse side effects. Drawing from the ancient discipline of yoga, along with modern understanding and methods from Energy Medicine, this book shows you how to be a maestro of your own energies, bringing your body, mind, and spirit into greater balance, health, and vitality."

DONNA EDEN AND DAVID FEINSTEIN
coauthors of *The Energies of Love*

"If you want to take your yoga practice—and your existence—out of the flat-lands and into the majestic peaks that form Energy Medicine Yoga, then read this book! Get ready for an exciting journey that will transform your practice, your perspective, and your life."

DONDI DAHLIN
author of the bestselling book *The Five Elements*

"Emerging science suggests that human health is not only linked to the function of the body but, more importantly, is found in what we cannot see—which is powerfully impacted by the energetic effect of what we think, see, and feel. This *is* Energy Medicine, and we must know it. *The Energy Medicine Yoga Prescription* is a must-read!"

DR. JOHN DOUILLARD, DC, CAP
founder of LifeSpa.com and author of *Eat Wheat*

"Drawing on insights from the Chinese Five Elements theory and the Vedic systems of yoga and Ayurveda, *The Energy Medicine Yoga Prescription* offers an interesting perspective on self-care. It will help you think in a different way about bringing health and balance into your life."

GARY KRAFTSOW
founder of the American Viniyoga Institute

"This is a beautiful book, rich with tools for a healthier lifestyle and a deepening of your yoga practice. Lauren writes in a clear and warm way that is easy to read and invites you into her eclectic collection of age-old remedies, health hints, recipes, and exercises."

ANGELA FARMER
free-flowing movement through yoga explorer

"As a professional athlete, I deal with a lot of pressure and nerves. *The Energy Medicine Yoga Prescription* has helped me realize how important it is to clear my energy field. We as human-spiritual beings have to take the time to clear our aura and energy field so we can radiate light and be a loving force."

JAMIE ANDERSON
Olympic gold medal snowboarder; yogi; activist

"If you are ready to explore the powerful dimensions of feeling, energy, and healing, *The Energy Medicine Yoga Prescription* will be your indispensable guide. You will learn invaluable tools to listen to the body's signals, to understand and communicate with the body not just for deeper yoga, but for a profoundly more healthy and joyous life."

EOIN FINN
founder of Blissology Yoga; author and cofacilitator
of Yoga + Mind Body Medicine courses

"It's high time someone correlated Energy Medicine with yoga. After all, both are designed to move energy through the body and the chakras for greater aliveness and well-being. Both are based on ancient, tried-and-true methods. Lauren Walker has done a great job of charting Five Elements theory, yoga, the meridian system, and many other wonderful tools to enter the state of union that yoga is all about."

ANODEA JUDITH, PHD
author of *Chakra Yoga, Wheels of Life,* and *Creating on Purpose*

"*The Energy Medicine Yoga Prescription* is a guide for the person who wants to increase their health and vitality and knows that the most effective path is one that combines physical, intellectual, and spiritual dimensions. The secret sauce to that outcome is through the energy system of the body, and Lauren Walker offers a multitude of easy-to-apply methods to affect that system through breath, diet, tapping, movement, gratitude, self-compassion, and much more."

CRAIG WEINER, DC
Emotional Freedom Techniques (EFT) international trainer; and
ALINA FRANK, EFT
international trainer and author of the bestselling
How to Want Sex Again: Rekindling Passion with EFT

"In *The Energy Medicine Yoga Prescription*, Lauren Walker pierces the superficiality of the yoga culture and shares powerful practices from the depths of ancient yogic traditions that will create a powerful impact on your health and healing."

JP SEARS
author of *How to Be Ultra Spiritual*

"A wonderful, pragmatic book illuminating the energy body and how to work with it for optimum health!"

ACHARYA SHUNYA
author of *Ayurveda Lifestyle Wisdom*

"Thrilled to see healing integrated into daily practice in this important guidebook. Donna Eden is a reliable source, and Lauren Walker has created a fabulous tool for transformation."

THORNTON STREETER, DSC
director of the Centre for Biofield Sciences and
founder of the Energy Medicine Exchange

"Connecting to our body's energy and eating healthy food is the path to healing. Lauren Walker's *The Energy Medicine Yoga Prescription* accomplishes this highly necessary and sometimes difficult relationship beautifully. Weaving her advanced knowledge of Energy Medicine through the practice of yoga is a divine therapeutic tool."

MARIE MANUCHEHRI
author of *Intuitive Self-Healing* and
How to Communicate with Your Spirit Guides

THE ENERGY MEDICINE YOGA PRESCRIPTION

Also by Lauren Walker

Energy Medicine Yoga: Amplify the Healing Power of Your Yoga Practice

LAUREN WALKER

THE ENERGY MEDICINE YOGA PRESCRIPTION

Learn five core practices
for hundreds of ailments

Discover three essential habits
for well-being

Activate your body's
natural healing intelligence

Create a powerful new vision
for health and happiness

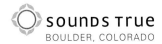
sounds true
BOULDER, COLORADO

Sounds True, Inc.
Boulder, CO 80306

Published 2017

Cover design by Rachael Murray
Book design by Beth Skelley
Cover and interior photos © Brooks Freehill

Printed in South Korea

Library of Congress Cataloging-in-Publication Data
Names: Walker, Lauren, author.
Title: The energy medicine yoga prescription / Lauren Walker.
Description: Boulder, CO : Sounds True, Inc., [2017] | Includes bibliographical references.
Identifiers: LCCN 2016051464 (print) | LCCN 2016051529 (ebook) |
    ISBN 9781622036615 (pbk.) | ISBN 9781622037506 (standard ebook) |
    ISBN 9781622037490 (enhanced ebook)
Subjects: LCSH: Hatha yoga. | Energy medicine. | Mind and body.
Classification: LCC RA781.7 .W346 2017 (print) | LCC RA781.7 (ebook) |
    DDC 613.7/046—dc23
LC record available at https://lccn.loc.gov/2016051464

10 9 8 7 6 5 4 3

This book would not have been possible without the generous support of Donna Eden, David Feinstein, and their school, Innersource. Their passion for teaching, sharing, and healing is unbounded, equaled only by their generosity. What they have given the world is an unprecedented path of healing, and with their blessings I am honored to adapt and promote their work through the lens of yoga. The Five Elements Body Ailments table, the Five Elements Mind Ailments table, and the Five Elements Self-Inventory have been adapted from the Innersource curriculum, with their generous permission.

Energy Medicine Yoga is backed by thousands of Innersource-trained Energy Medicine practitioners all over the world. If you are dealing with something beyond the scope of self-practice, please contact one of them at Innersource.net. If you are interested in becoming a certified Innersource practitioner or EMYoga teacher, please see the resource section at the back of the book.

For You, for healing

Contents

Prescriptions for Your Health

Be the Mountain; Be the Skier

By my third winter downhill skiing, I was really learning how to drop in. In yoga, "dropping in" means to let go of the chattering mind and let yourself be taken over by the immediacy and intimacy of your practice. In skiing it means to go over the edge, down into the bowl, down into the gravity of your chosen run with complete abandon and trust.

The two are nearly identical.

I was finally learning to trust my body, to trust my gear, to trust my instincts. The snow is different every day: fresh, deep, sticky, graupelly, chicken-heady, icy, powder—the list to describe the consistency of the snow goes on and on. Then there's the ambient weather. Is it actively snowing? Sleeting? Raining? Graupelling? Sunny? Cloudy? Foggy?

We go down the same mountain, over all its flanks, day after day, hour after hour. The repetition builds confidence and strength. But there is also pure joy. The body goes into a joy response that many people liken to orgasm—simply by sliding down a hill covered in snow.

Energy Medicine Yoga—the marriage of Energy Medicine with a tantra-based yoga practice—has the same possibility and the same parallel. We come to our yoga mat day after day, hour after hour. Our energy, like the snow, is also changeable; every day it's different. But we do the same moves again and again. There isn't anywhere to get to. There's no prize at the end for the most downward dogs. It is simply the moment that is sublime. It is like coming home to a feeling of goodness in our own bodies.

This is the important part: We need to feel good in our lives and in our bodies just as we are right now. We need to know how to self-soothe and how to heal. So many of us go for the outside stimuli of drugs, alcohol, shopping, sugar, or sex when we're uncomfortable, bored, or tired. If we're sick, we go for outside cures: pills, surgery, radiation. But we must learn how to simply and effectively take care of ourselves from the inside to be healthy and happy.

In my first book, *Energy Medicine Yoga*, I used the metaphor of grooming the ski slopes on the mountain as being equivalent to grooming the energies that run the body. We usually think of grooming in terms of our teeth, hair, makeup, and overall self-care. But like grooming the ski runs, we groom our body's energies—the meridians, the chakras, the aura. We fluff them all up; get them smoothed out, cleaned, and organized; and off we go. Just as the runs on the mountain are groomed each night before the next day's skiers arrive, our energy systems need daily grooming.

Now let's extend the metaphor. Once you go off into your life, you *become* the skier on the mountain. You are now taking these energy systems with you because they *are* you, and they are constantly changing. Being the mountain, you must come into stillness, calm, and solidity, having your energy work to help you ground and center. Being the skier, you must come into movement, the flow of life and experiences, and have your energy maintain its balancing work, no matter what is going on.

Each of us is really a moving ball of energy, fields and lines, vortexes and swirls, all zooming around our central core, and we're moving through the world, which is full of millions of similar but different energy systems all zooming around. We tend to see these energy systems and ourselves as fixed figures. But really we are just zooming bits of information and light. It's all very Jetsony, except its invisible and its real.

Energy Medicine Yoga taught how to groom the mountain, the physical structure of the body. In this book, you're going to learn how to be the skier—how to be the energetic structure, how to master the art of moving through the constantly changing world without falling down, ejecting from both of your skis, losing your hat, mittens, goggles, and poles—what is called in ski language a "yard sale!" Another ski phrase that is helpful is this: it's all about the recovery! Sometimes what the mountain throws at you—what life throws at you—is too much to handle. How you negotiate and recover from it is essential to maintaining your health and sanity. If you ski up to a cliff, you might not want to launch off and go sailing thirty feet into the air. You need to know how to sidestep around it, how to sideslip down the icy shoot, how to bring yourself to safety. When you start to lose your balance because you're leaning too far forward or too far back, you need the inner awareness, strength, and skill to bring your body back over your skis so you don't wreck—on the slopes, or in your life!

In yoga, we are constantly uniting opposites: yin and yang, extension and contraction, the individual soul and the eternal Soul. Because we are both the physical structure and the energetic structure, we must be able to affect change on both of these levels. It isn't an either-or proposition, as this book will show, but a both-and. We are both the physical structure and the energetic structure. Neither is more important, but the energetic structure is often ignored for lack of information, knowledge, or tools to access it.

The goal is to be both the mountain and the skier. As the mountain, you have your underlying energy systems working at their best. As the skier, you navigate your life and are able to handle anything it throws at you. You can recover and thrive no matter what comes your way by understanding how to work with energy in movement.

PART 1

Mind

Understanding Energy

∞

Your thoughts and beliefs are the single most important indicator of your state of health. . . . Your beliefs and thoughts are wired into your biology. They become your cells, tissues, and organs. There's no supplement, no diet, no medicine, and no exercise regimen that can compare with the power of your thoughts and beliefs. That's the very first place you need to look when anything goes wrong with your body.

CHRISTIANE NORTHRUP, MD
Goddesses Never Age

1

Energy and Mind-Body Health

Everything in the universe is energy vibrating at different frequencies. If you want to affect the physical matter that is your body and the invisible matter that is your mind and your soul—in the most efficient and powerful way—you must learn how to work with your own personal energy. This book is a guide to help you do just that. Specifically, you will learn how to work with and balance the energy systems that make up your body and that you experience indirectly by their effects.

Because most of us don't see energy, it can be hard to understand how it is the most powerful force in our lives. But we generally don't understand how our cell phones work, or our TVs, or the physics behind an airplane, and yet every day we use these technologies, completely trusting.

If things in your life are out of whack or if you are experiencing a health crisis of any kind—mental, physical, or spiritual—you are experiencing energy that is out of balance. Even if you are not in crisis but you feel overwhelmed, tired, anxious, melancholy, or rageful, you are experiencing energy that is out of balance. And even if you feel great most of the time but sometimes you feel completely off (depression strikes, you're going through a period of doubt, or you just broke your leg), your underlying energy at that moment is out of balance.

When you are in balance and flow, your body and mind are working well, synergistically and coherently—meaning the least amount of effort is expended to accomplish all the tasks necessary for living and thriving. You are in resonance with yourself and your life path. You may feel tired after a long bike ride or a long day of work, but you fall asleep easily, your body rebuilds, and the next day you feel good again. If this is not the case, your energy is out of balance.

Many self-help books talk about body, mind, and spirit. But there is a fourth layer of being, the layer of energy. This whole book is essentially an explanation of how to access and use this fourth layer in the context of the other three. It may seem strange to call it another layer, since it is in fact what the other three are made up of. But if we don't separate it out and talk about it as a distinct entity, we risk losing the true and inherent power of energy. If you have a broken leg, cancer, eczema, depression, attention-deficit disorder, unremitting sadness, or deep angst, you might say you don't really care about energy—you want to heal your leg, your mind, or your soul. Yet here is the single most important thing to understand: *it is the energy that needs to heal first.* Only then can everything else heal.

All successful medical interventions and psychotherapies work at the energetic level, intentionally or unwittingly, along with whatever they are consciously targeting. Shifting the energies is the most direct way of targeting a problem. So even if you can't see energy, this book will teach you how to sense it, work with it, understand it, change it, and align with it.

The first part of the book explains the basis of EMYoga. You'll learn how your mind and emotions affect your health and how you can bring them into healthier alignment with simple techniques. You'll learn how to feel your own energy and how to energy test, giving you an invaluable tool for diagnosing problems and making healthy choices. You'll get a basic description of the energy systems that make up the body, and an in-depth view of the Five Elements system, the energy system around which the healing practices are designed.

The main practice section of the book, part 2, gives you the Essential EMYoga practice for health and well-being, as well as a full video available online. This is your baseline practice to start getting your energies working for you. There is also a list of body and mind ailments in two Five Elements tables (see pages 52–64) to help you find the practice that will help resolve any specific ailment you may have. Then there are five main healing practices, one for each element. Each element has a brief description followed by the EMYoga practice to balance it, along with accompanying photographs and at times links to videos.

Part 3 ties together ways to balance many other facets of life off the yoga mat. It includes the three most important Ayurvedic techniques that will change your life right now. In part 3, we'll also cover EMYoga practices for diet and nutrition, body image, and how to truly love yourself, the cornerstone of all healing.

These outcomes may sound like a lot to promise, but the truth is, once you start working with energy, you see the infinite possibilities and the remarkable results.

The beautiful and most powerful thing is that working with the energies of the body is quite simple. You don't have to be able to do a one-armed handstand or sit in a full lotus. If you can breathe, you can do EMYoga. At the same time, it isn't a quick fix. This isn't a pill, a cream, or a tincture. This isn't chemotherapy, chelation, or reflexology. This is a series of tools, practices, and wisdoms that you can bring into your life to make your life better.

Bringing together two enormous fields of study creates a more enormous field of study. But don't get overwhelmed. It also gets infinitely smaller. That's how energy, and nature, works. Self-similar at all levels. The beauty of this is once you understand the concepts and you learn a few of the levers and pulleys, you can affect the biggest area with the least amount of effort. The practices are simple. Start to do one or two of them, and see how your energy shifts and your day seems to open up and become longer and less cluttered. This book is meant to be a resource to last you many years, it isn't essential to learn all of the practices at once. Take your time, dip in and out, see the benefits unfold, and then go back and learn another layer.

There is repetition in yoga, as in skiing, as in life. We do the same things over and over again. This can lead to boredom, or joy; this can lead to bad habits, or help deepen your skills. Much depends on your outlook, and your intentions. Some concepts in this book will be repeated too, to help you understand new ideas by seeing them more than once. As you continue to practice, day after day, clear goals will lead you up the path of mastery instead of into a rut. I like to remind myself of this with the words of the brilliant musician Prince: "There's joy in repetition."

The magic and complexity of your body makes your iPhone look like a Fisher-Price toy. The body can do things that science still cannot explain, like differentiate cells and heal itself miraculously. But when things go wrong, it can be challenging to know where to look to fix them. For far too long, we looked at the body mechanistically, like a car. We replaced parts. Only recently have we begun to look at the body holistically, understanding that every part affects every other part. Your emotions affect your organs; your organs affect your emotions; your thoughts affect your physiology—everything affects everything else. And underneath all of that, the substrate on which your physical, mental, and emotional being rests is energy. It not only rests in energy, it *is* energy. You are at one level no more than a vibrating, pulsing wave form that is moving slowly enough to appear solid. This might be hard to wrap your head around, but I'm going to show you ways to work with these invisible energies, to feel them and transform them so they become much more than a metaphor or a strange concept. Learning to work with your energies will connect you with the deepest realms of your being. You will not only understand how and why things go wrong when they do, but how to bring them back to right. To have the life you truly want and deserve, you have to heal the issues that are holding you back. Some of these challenges are physical, some emotional, some spiritual. But all of them are rooted in energy.

The Magic of Energy Medicine Yoga

Energy follows certain rules:

1   Energy wants to move.

2   Energy needs space to move.

3   Energy follows particular patterns in the body.

4   The two most important energy patterns are moving forward and crossing from one side of the body to the other.

5   The root cause of any ailment is energy not moving forward and/or crossing over.

When I became an EM (Energy Medicine) practitioner, I worked with clients who were lying down on my table. I'd help them correct their energy imbalances, give them some techniques to do at home, and then watch them get healthier as their issues improved, resolved, and healed. I would do all of these techniques on myself too because there weren't any other EM practitioners in my small town.

I'd also been teaching yoga, and I started combining EM and yoga together, simply to be more efficient, and was surprised at the benefits I felt personally. When I began introducing these concepts in the classes I was teaching at Norwich University, I was blown away by the results. Either practice on its own is powerful, as any EM client or yoga student can tell you. What surprised me was how much more powerful it was to put them together. This is because of the rules of energy. With the yoga practice, we are giving our energy room and space to move. With the EM practice, we are guiding the energy in the directions it wants and needs to flow. With the repetition of the combined practices of EM and yoga, we help the energy to repattern and remain in these new, beneficial flows. The EM student gets the physical benefits of moving and opening the body. The yoga student gets the awareness of how and where to move energy. Putting the practices together, we get a healing paradigm that offers results that seem magical.

Once your energy is working for and with you, almost anything is possible. Teachers and students who have practiced yoga for years suddenly start shifting things that were stuck. Chronic pain, digestive complaints, depression, relationship struggles, hopelessness, pulled muscles, sleep disorders, indecision—these are just some of the issues that get resolved by students who have often tried every other kind of alternative practice with no result. They start to practice Energy Medicine Yoga (EMYoga), and abracadabra! Magic happens.

The energy systems we'll be working with (explained in chapter 2) have been identified in many healing and spiritual traditions. Eden Energy Medicine, as taught by healing pioneer and my mentor Donna Eden, teaches about nine energy systems in the body that are vital for health and well-being. Donna's genius was creating techniques for working with them all together, exactly how they work in the body. EMYoga takes those same concepts and those same energy systems and weaves them into a yoga practice.

EMYoga is a tantra-based practice. The Sanskrit word *tantra* means to weave and to stretch toward. More broadly it also refers to systematic techniques for achieving a particular outcome. The yoga part of EMYoga is grounded in a practice with emphasis on various techniques to help you accept your innate perfection and from there transform into, or stretch toward, becoming your best self.

When I first started studying tantra yoga, I was amazed at all the things involved that seemed to have nothing to do with my idea of "yoga"—things like Vedic astrology, gemology, and aromatherapy, as well as things like gratitude, journaling, and rituals. But as I've come to understand the deeper meaning and power of yoga, it all makes perfect sense. If we want to reach the goal of ultimate union with ourselves, and with the divine, we need to master more than just the physical body.

In EMYoga you'll learn asana practices (physical postures) that incorporate poses and moves to access your underlying energy. Some of the poses look similar to yoga poses you may already be familiar with. Others will be complete departures from standard yoga and are used to influence specific flows of energy. You'll use the electromagnetic energy of your own body, often with your hands, to affect the energy in your body—sort of like those old Wooly Willy games where you pull the magnet around to draw features on a face with iron filings.

The power and comprehensive practices of EMYoga incorporate pranayama (breathing practices), meditation, visualization, journaling, EFT (Emotional Freedom Technique) tapping, nutrition, diet, body image, and belief systems. The beauty of energy work is that it translates into every facet of your life—from what, how, and when you eat to how you think and how you feel about your body, mind, and life. It only starts on the mat. EMYoga touches every area of your life because energy touches every area of your life. The result of this practice is a deep love, appreciation, and acceptance of yourself just as you are now. This is one of the most powerful takeaways: self-love. From that place, all healing, transformation, contentment, and peace are possible. Being in flow with life, having gratitude for your very existence and experiences, joy at your abilities, compassion for others—these are the gifts life has to offer and the fruits of your EMYoga practice.

Your Personal Prescription for Health

℞, the shorthand for *prescription*, is the doodle that a caregiver writes at the top of a list, telling the patient "Take this!" ℞ is itself shorthand for the word *recipe*, which means "take" in Latin, as in "Take this medicine." In medieval times, ℞ was a list of ingredients or activities the patient was to imbibe or undertake to resolve a stated ailment. Healing cures or therapies given to people were recipes for their lives.

The practices in this book are meant to be your own personal recipe, your prescription for healing and empowering you to live your best life. Your personal recipe is a prescription to stay healthy as well as for healing if you're sick. If your life is full of challenges and obstacles, whether physical, mental, emotional, or spiritual, you can use this book to find a recipe to transform your disparate parts into a healthy and balanced whole. Both ancient Chinese Medicine and Ayurveda (the medical arm of yoga) hold the tenet that balance is the holy grail of healing. The body will do its own miraculous healing if its systems are in balance.

The Essential EMYoga practice, presented in part 2, is a thirty-minute routine that includes the main poses and energy-clearing techniques to help you balance your body. If you have a specific issue you're dealing with, you can then move on to one of the Five Element practices that go deeper into the work of each specific element. You devise your own recipe from the list of ingredients offered in this book. The ingredients are many and varied: asanas, breath work, food choices, body-care protocols, journaling, topics to think and dream about, gratitude, and tapping. You will create a unique recipe based on the particular outcome you're looking for, and you'll adjust the ℞ as you experience changes.

Throughout the book, there are many suggestions of things you can do, outside of your asana practice, that can help your energy. These are marked with the ℞ symbol. These are add-on practices to support your healing. Try them out; if they resonate with you, add them to your personal EMYoga prescription.

The first step is learning to work directly with your own energy. This is much easier and more accessible than you could ever have imagined. Your energy is like a thumbprint; it is unique to you. This means that how you heal, how you thrive, how you grow and change is also unique to you.

Once you tap into your energy systems, cultivating a daily practice with consistency and devotion is the most important thing you can do to live healthfully and heal disease. It isn't what you do every once in a while that can harm or heal; it is what you do most of the time. And that is true with your energy systems as well. Energy moves in patterns, has memory, and evolves, which can help keep you stuck or help release you. But release only happens when you start to consistently introduce and practice new energy patterns.

If your body is showing dis-ease or your mind is showing dis-ease, a series of events brought you to this point. When you introduce a consistent EMYoga practice, you start to see shifts in these dis-ease patterns. Once your practice becomes a part of your daily life, you'll have the skill set to detect and resolve issues at the start before they get serious.

It is also important to identify what your goals and obstacles are and what difficulties you are currently seeking help for. In other words, why did you pick up this book? Oftentimes, crafting the question is the most difficult part to finding the perfect answer. Once you go through the ailment lists (pages 52–64) and take the Five Elements Self-Inventory (page 39), you'll have a map to the practices that will serve you best right now.

As you read through the book, or flip through it, the things that jump out at you or attract your attention are the things to focus on. Trust your intuition, and trust your own energy to steer you toward creating your own perfect recipe that serves you right now. Listening to your inner guides will become your fail-safe tool to finding the answers to the questions presenting themselves.

In the next chapters you'll begin learning about the power of energy and the different systems that make up EMYoga. Use a highlighter or a pen, or your own journal, to start making notes on the things that draw your attention. Your notes will help guide you and ensure that this system works specifically for you.

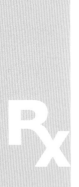

JOURNALING

When you start any new practice, it is helpful to take notes on your journey. Otherwise, even things that you initially think are remarkable and unforgettable will soon be hard to recall. I always ask students at the beginning of practice how they feel and then again at the end of practice. If you are starting your study of EMYoga with a particular issue to resolve, it is helpful to write down how changes happen and when. It is also helpful to chart your progress and to take notes on things you like or dislike, areas of difficulty or challenge, and areas of the body or mind that are sore, stiff, or challenged.

LEARN THIS MOST IMPORTANT PRACTICE
AND BREAK IN YOUR JOURNAL

Try doing the Wake Up (see page 78) every day for thirty days. Write down in your journal the date and time of day you did it with a check mark or a smiley face. This practice helps you see how easily you can commit to yourself, even in a small way, and also see what changes that commitment brings.

If you are working with a particular health challenge, sometimes you can find the underlying emotion of a physical complaint by doing some stream-of-consciousness writing, where you simply allow yourself to write without thinking or editing. This is a way to tap into the unconscious mind.

I suggest you have your journal with you during all of your practices so you can take notes when something arises that you want to remember. For example, if you're doing the wood practice, you might write down the physical challenges you have in the wood element. Write down the things you're angry about. What would be a way to move from anger to assertiveness? Can you find ways to let the anger motivate you to action that is helpful and powerful? At the end of your practice, you can see what came up during your practice and meditation. Did you feel a shift in the areas of anger? What solutions presented themselves to you? Did you feel a shift in the physical areas governed by wood?

At times, you may even forget that you were afflicted with something when it resolves, and it can be helpful to look back and see that you did indeed have X or Y, but your body healed it. These moments are incredibly powerful. If you are dealing with a more serious issue, tracking the changes and interventions that you've used can also be empowering.

Another thing to use your journal for is doodling. Drawing connects the hemispheres of your brain and creates new neural links. You can doodle figure eights to increase them in your fields (the most powerful pattern to have in your fields). You can also doodle the Triskele and the Five Element Wheel (see page 44). Doodling shifts you out of linear thinking into the quantum realm—the place you make real leaps in terms of change. It is these leaps that are called "miracles" or "magic." It is connecting with Einstein's "spooky action at a distance"—and it is not only attainable, it is learnable and replicable.

Use your journal as your own personal EMYoga book, and let yourself be free enough to discover the power it has for you personally.

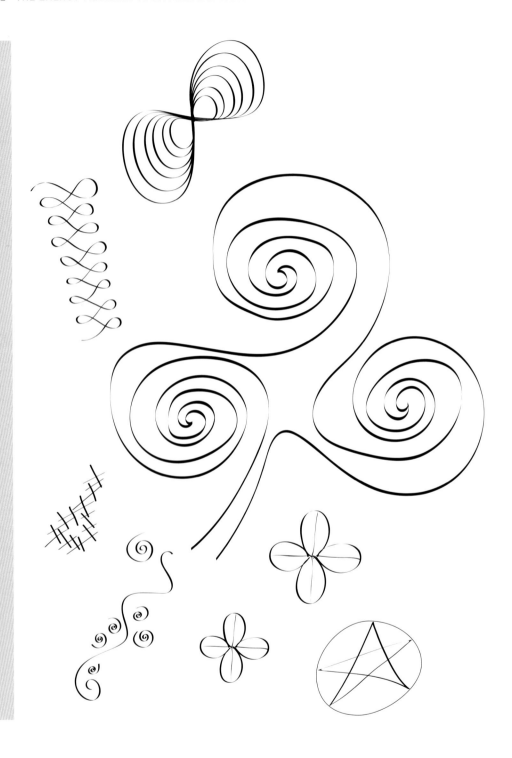

Healing versus Curing

As you start to go deeper into this book, especially if you are suffering from an illness, it is vitally important that you understand the difference between "healing" and "curing." Matthew Sanford, author of the book *Waking*, is one of the leading teachers of adaptive yoga and is a paraplegic. He responds elegantly about this in an interview with *Yoga Digest*:

> I think that so much of our culture is fixated on healing as a reversal of condition. Anyone who has lived through trauma knows you can never go home. It's never going to be the same, and that's okay. I'm never going to walk again—does that mean healing is done for me? Does that mean the only healing possible is for me to have a good attitude about being paralyzed? Absolutely not! What yoga creates is the conditions for people to heal in unexpected ways if they can just look beyond healing as curing.[1]

It is sometimes impossible to understand the path of your life, especially when it takes an unexpected turn toward illness, disease, trauma, or loss. You cast about for answers, build stories to explain your new life, and move forward as best you can. What EMYoga offers in the face of these huge challenges is the ability to slow down, tune in, and understand the body and mind in a different way. Some challenges can be reversed; some diseases and conditions can heal or go dormant. There are many techniques in EMYoga that can help you transform the despair of your challenge into acceptance and understanding so that you can thrive in your life, as Matthew has, instead of just survive. It's also important to understand that nothing is going to take away the experience you've undergone. But that doesn't mean that healing isn't an option. There are many ways to heal and many ways to live your life that are sometimes different from what you'd planned or hoped for. This resiliency is in fact a huge part of healing.

How Your Mind Affects Your Health

In Christiane Northrup's wonderful book *Goddesses Never Age*, she writes about an important finding from a longitudinal study of nuns begun in 1986: "Autopsies showed that the nuns who relished life and showed no signs of dementia had just as many plaques in their brains as the less vivacious nuns whose dementia was apparent before they died."[2] That's right—both groups had the exact same amount of plaque in the brain, the plaque that many scientists believe is the underlying cause of Alzheimer's. Yet those nuns who experienced joy, creativity, and love of life never showed any signs of dementia. How is that possible? If we look only at the physiological evidence, we might conclude it isn't possible, or call it a miracle. But if we look at the mind as transcending the body, it makes much more sense. Our mind affects us more than anything else except energy.

Ideas such as the placebo effect—cures that happen simply because we *believe* they will—are often dismissed as anomalies, but the truth is, the placebo effect proves that our mind is more powerful than our body; it proves that our mind has choices and is not simply mechanistic.[3]

One of the strangest and most intriguing instances of the power of the mind is the documentation of patients with multiple personality disorders. Deepak Chopra, MD, writes of one such instance in *Perfect Health*. A young child had an extreme allergic reaction to orange juice, resulting in sores all over his skin. When another of the child's personalities was present in his mind-body, there was no allergic reaction or physiological response.[4] This points to the fact that the mind has a "choice" about what it reacts to and can change its "mind" instantaneously. Thoughts supersede the chemical interactions of the body. In the case of the young patient, his thoughts were unconscious thoughts. If they could be brought to consciousness, they would be unstoppable in their healing capacity.

One way the mind can literally remap itself is with visualization practices. In the book *The Brain's Way of Healing*, Canadian psychiatrist Norman Doidge gives clinical evidence of people with extreme and chronic pain who had been relegated to ingesting powerful painkillers for their whole lives. Doidge profiled Michael Moskowitz, a psychiatrist-turned-pain specialist, who taught his clients intense visualization practices and found that they could actually change the structure and outcomes that the brain created. He reduced and eliminated chronic pain by having his patients shrink their pain receptors and transform the brain's maps and experience of pain with the power of their own thinking.[5]

Visualization is one of the tools we'll use to move energy through the body. Many studies attest to its power. Groups as diverse as elite athletes and people with paralysis use visualization practices with incredible results.

My own personal experience of healing with my mind came from *Healing Back Pain* by John E. Sarno, MD. Sarno links all back pain to undigested anger, and since I started doing the practice he recommended, after years of chiropractic adjustments, I have not had another back issue.

These are all instances of the conscious mind working to heal the body. But what about the unconscious mind? We saw the young boy with multiple personalities in a battle between his conscious and unconscious mind determine what manifests in his body. A placebo works by unifying the conscious mind's beliefs with the unconscious mind's habits. Getting those two aligned is probably the single most life-transforming thing you can do. Bruce H. Lipton, PhD, author of *The Biology of Belief* and *The Honeymoon Effect*, offers clear and simple insight into the power of the unconscious that runs our lives.

The conscious mind is what you're thinking right now. It is your ego, your sense of self, your decision maker. It is also the creative mind, the more advanced part of you that can *respond* to stimuli rather than just react by instinct. It is the part of you that holds your dreams and desires. Your unconscious mind is the programming that runs everything else—it runs 95 percent of your life and actions. It is where your habits are held. Your unconscious mind was programmed when you were a child, up until about the age of seven. The things that come easily to you, without thinking, without effort, were programmed well into your unconscious. If you heard your parents argue about a lack of money as you grew up, you'll likely run that program as an adult, and chances are you'll struggle with money too.[6]

The beautiful thing is, you can rewrite your unconscious programming. This means accessing the unconscious mind and inserting new, positive programs that align with the desires of your conscious mind.

The reason breathing practices (pranayama, page 69) are so important in yoga is that your breath is a direct link between your conscious and unconscious mind, and shifting one shifts the other. Tapping (page 32), journaling, automatic writing, and vocalizations are other tools for shifting these patterns. EMYoga is designed to unite these opposing forces so that you are in true alignment with your soul's deepest desires, your highest purpose, and your best life.

The only thing as powerful as the mind is energy, and another of the goals of this book is to bring those two elements into union, another uniting of seeming opposites. It's incredibly important to realize that you hold the key to healing inside yourself. Your beliefs and ideas affect you more than any other single thing on the planet. And your beliefs are tied inextricably with the fields of energy that underpin your body.

How Energy Affects Your Health

The science behind the mind-body connection has finally reached the mainstream. There is now solid research that connects our emotions, our levels of stress and joy, and other mind states directly to physical issues.

Research on the power of subtle energy to affect the body is still in its infancy, but it is building, and in another few years, my hope is that the understanding of energy's ability to affect change in the body will be mainstream. Techniques such as acupuncture, which works on the meridians (one of our energy systems), and Reiki (a hands-on healing technique) have been studied and documented for their beneficial effects. More and more people are finding relief from their challenges in ways that would have been entirely dismissed just a few years ago.

James L. Oschman, PhD, has spent a lifetime quantifying how Energy Medicine works. He gives us the science of how the physical body is connected seamlessly to the energetic body through our fascia. The importance of this information is that it explains how things such as acupuncture, acupressure, and the many other techniques of EMYoga work. Our bodies are completely interconnected energetically so that when you apply energy to one area of the body, it is instantaneously transmitted to the entire body.

Here is a brief excerpt from a talk he gave to our advanced class in 2013 in Phoenix, Arizona, at Innersource, Donna Eden's school of Energy Medicine:

> The living matrix is a system that extends throughout the
> body and physically connects all of the parts together. It is
> the one living system that touches all of the other systems.

> It interpenetrates and surrounds all organs, muscles, bones, and nerve fibers . . . the components of this matrix are electronic semiconductors. . . . This means that the electrons in the proteins and other molecules are not confined to the chemical bonds that hold the system together but are free to move around, conveying energy and information throughout the organism. The quantum physics description is that the electrons are delocalized. Quantum physics and semiconduction are at the foundation of Energy Medicine.

According to Oschman, this living matrix, also called the extracellular matrix, is essentially the connective tissue or collagen that runs through and around every system in the body. It "exerts specific and important influences upon cellular dynamics, just as much as hormones or neurotransmitters."[7]

Another invisible system of energy that affects the body is the morphic field. First postulated in the early 1900s to explain the growth of embryos, the hypothesis was expanded upon by the contemporary biologist Rupert Sheldrake, PhD, into an explanation of the organizing principle not only for biological structures but for all things in nature, from crystals to cells to human communities. The morphic field hypothesis suggests that everything in the physical world develops and organizes itself in resonance with preexisting invisible fields. To make it even more interesting, these morphic (literally "form-giving") fields themselves evolve over time, providing a unique perspective for understanding what Sheldrake calls the "habits of nature."[8]

Donna had long observed a field that organizes and influences the development of the body's energy systems. This field is a layer within the aura, the energy field that surrounds and protects the body. When she met Dr. Sheldrake and heard him explain his theory of "morphic resonance," it was a bingo moment for her. Sheldrake's explanations corresponded perfectly with this particular layer of the aura, its influence on the body's energies, and the subsequent influence of the body's energy systems on the body's physical structures and their functioning. Like Sheldrake's morphic fields, this "morphic" layer of the aura evolves over time and is responsible for the habits of our energies, both those that serve us and those that don't. Once we are aware of this field and gain some tools to access it, we enter into the realm of applied morphic resonance, the ability to transform our physical and energetic systems by way of these fields. A number of simple, tactile ways to work with our morphic fields to change habitual patterns in our energies, our bodies, and even our thinking and behavior have been innovated (one of these is presented on page 34).

Morphic fields help explain why it can be so difficult to affect change, as they are designed to conserve habits, a principle of evolution. They also help us understand our interconnectivity with each other and with our world. Groups that are similar hold a similar resonance, and all members of that group, according to this hypothesis, are affected when a critical mass of a group's members learn a new task. This corresponds with the yogic tenet "Heal yourself; heal the world."

Morphic resonance explains why what you do in the world matters for the collective. Individual energy has a huge effect. It gathers. It forms patterns, systems, and habits. For instance, a relatively small number of people who are intent on a shared purpose can change seemingly intransigent structures in the world. That is why mass changes in world dynamics are called "movements." People moving together, bringing their habits together, increase the strength of the field and this then reverberates to the group.

Peaceful protests are a potent example of people moving together toward a common good. If you feel despair at the challenges of our current world, you can take faith in the knowledge that energy can indeed shift and that your individual energy can contribute to that shift. How each of us lives becomes how the world lives.

Patterns can be difficult to change. We see that when we try to break self-defeating habits. Changing a habit requires conscious intention, repetition, and willpower. But habits can and do change. Whether we are trying to change the habits of the world or the habits of our body, they require the same types of intervention. And although it may seem difficult, if there is enough of a critical mass, the change of the few can energetically pave the way for change in the many. While this may seem like a magical explanation, if we adopt the lens of morphic resonance, it explains many of the body's miraculous healing capacities. Mastering the invisible forces that impact us every day turns us into magicians of our health and vitality. The sooner we embrace this, the sooner we can start to work the magic in our lives that we so deeply crave. Energy and magic are intimately intertwined. Both invisible; both powerful.

The body has an innate, built-in capacity for healing. In fact, that is what the body wants to do and spends most of its time doing. After digestion, the biggest thing the body does is rebuild itself—cleaning, organizing, and eliminating toxins. The body knows how to heal, and mostly what we need to do is stop inhibiting that natural function. Andrew Weil, MD, a pioneer in the field of integrative medicine, summarizes this concept perfectly in his bestselling book *Spontaneous Healing*:

- Healing is an inherent capacity of life. DNA has within it all the information needed to manufacture enzymes to repair itself.

- The healing system operates continuously and is always on call.

- The healing system has a diagnostic capability; it can recognize damage.

- The healing system can remove damaged structure and replace it with normal structure.

- The healing system not only acts to neutralize the effects of serious injury . . . it also directs the ordinary, moment-to-moment corrections that maintain normal structure and function. . . .

- Healing is spontaneous.[9]

When your energies are organized and guided on the paths that optimize them, your body can take over and heal, giving you the power you need to be able to live your life the way you want.

To Change, You Have to Change

If you really want to change something in your life, you have to do the work to get there. A new habit takes time to create. You must practice. If you want to change your life, your path, or your health, you have to change the activities that brought you to where you currently are.

Change happens in the resting moments, in savasana, in the still points, called the *cesura*, the stop in the music, the held suspension of all quantum potential. Change happens when you stop. This is crucial to remember as you're doing this work and actively tracking your changes. Energy can shift instantly, but if you want to change longstanding patterns—physical, emotional, or spiritual—you have to change the underlying patterns of energy. You have to stop the detrimental energy patterns and start new health-supporting patterns. Those longstanding detrimental patterns are habits that your body resists changing. It requires repetition, willpower, and the intelligent application of energy to bring about real change.

Many of us need to stop the crazy rushing around and come into stillness, but the flip side of stillness is lethargy. In our culture we have busy minds, but oftentimes our bodies sit in chairs, cars, and couches all day. We need to shift this and get our bodies moving and still our minds.

START TO CHANGE: START SMALL

Do the Wake Up (page 78). Drive a different way to work. Order a different thing off the menu. Say yes when you would have said no. Say no when you would have said yes.

If you're struggling with a serious illness or dis-ease, you must often change many things at once. Look to your diet, your belief systems, your physical practices. If you're quite ill, and especially if you have an autoimmune illness, you must even look to changing where you live. Most modern homes are built with powerful toxins that can make you sick. If you want to get well, you might have to change everything. Once you embrace the power of change, it becomes less frightening, and can even be exciting. *To change, you have to change* seems so obvious. But it is often the most obvious that is the most difficult.

A NOTE ON CANCER AND
OTHER SERIOUS ILLNESSES

Cancer is one of the most terrifying diagnoses a person can get. An estimated 40 percent of people will get cancer in their lifetime,[10] but unfortunately there is no consensus on cause or cure. Our current choices of chemotherapy and radiation are extremely violent to the body and have a limited success rate. In fact, in a poll of 118 physicians, all cancer experts, nearly every one said they would not undergo such drastic treatment (radiation and chemotherapy) if they received a cancer diagnosis.[11] Western medicine is now identifying cancer as an immune system disease and looking at activating the patient's own immune system to counter the cancer.

Cancer is a holistic disease, not a mechanistic disease. There are many varied and result-oriented approaches to cancer all over the world. There is incredible promise with endocannabinoid therapy.[12] There are treatments of diet, cleansing, and Ayurvedic protocols, and much cutting-edge alternative research, particularly in Europe, including the controversial but compelling theories of German New Medicine.[13] Many of these therapies have been shown to be powerful against this disease.

If cancer is something that has entered your life, the first course of treatment is this: Do Not Lose Hope. There are many resources out there (some listed at the back of the book). A healthy body has cancer cells in it every day, and the immune system of a healthy body can eradicate these cells. We have the ability to cure ourselves of even this most disturbing phenomenon.

The practices in this book will support and help transform the underlying energies of any disease. These techniques work well, and often miraculously. However, it is also important to note that disease patterns and their resulting physical expression take many forms and may require many things to bring them under control. Sometimes, especially when dealing with something serious, we need the intervention of someone else to help us shift our energy. The beauty of EMYoga is that it is the only yoga system in the world

with a built-in health-care system behind it—thousands of certified EM practitioners around the world who are trained in this detailed, specific, and powerful work. If you find that your energy isn't shifting and you need more help, please contact a practitioner (see the resource section in back of book). Also keep in mind that if you are suffering from a serious illness, seek the attention of a qualified medical practitioner to help you navigate the confusing fields of help available both mainstream and alternative.

Working with Your Energy

Energy is subtle, but not as subtle as you may think. The first step to experiencing your own energy, so you can see results in your health and life right away, is to have an awareness of the energy systems in your body.

Here are the eight energy systems that we work with in EMYoga:

Meridians   energy pathways that run up and down the body, including along the arms and legs; these paths run deep inside the body and at points come close to the surface of the skin, forming acupuncture or acupressure points

Chakras   spiraling swirls of energy that spin outward and inward from seven main locations along the central line of the body, from the pubic bone to the crown of the head

Radiant Circuits   paths of energy that run around the body, back and front; unlike meridians on fixed pathways, Radiant Circuits travel wherever their healing energy is needed—these are the energies of healing and joy

Electrics   points on the body where the electrical component of all the energy systems is accessed

Aura   the field of energy that surrounds and protects the physical body

Celtic Weave   the outermost layer of the aura filled with geometric shapes, including the powerful figure eight crossover pattern of health

Triple Warmer   a superhero meridian that controls the immune system, the fight-flight-freeze response, as well as the distribution of energy, heat, and moisture throughout the body; it can also evolve into a Radiant Circuit, empowering and strengthening our life path

The Five Elements   the system that speaks with, influences, and unites all the energy systems and for that reason is the one used to create the healing practices in this book

Listening and Talking to Your Body

Your body talks to you in many ways. It talks in dreams, intuitions, and emotions. It talks by way of pain and other physical sensations that are often ignored until the body has to find stronger means to get your attention. Physically we talk back to the body by tapping, holding, weaving, massaging, and stretching. One of the main energetic "languages" of the body is pulse. Every cell pulses. Your heart beats, your blood pulses through your veins, your digestion works in a series of pulses, and your energy systems pulse with their positive and negative ionic charges. So one way to speak to and with your body is by "pulsing" with it, or tapping. Some ways we mentally speak to the body are with our thoughts and inner voices, imagination and visualization.

When I asked one of my student teachers what she thought was the most important thing about EMYoga, she said that in all of her other yoga trainings, she had heard the cues to "listen to the body, listen to the breath, and then use what you hear to help you move out from the body into the world." But she also said that those ideas had seemed merely conceptual until she studied EMYoga, which gave her the tools to listen to and hear the body's signals and interpret their meaning. More than that, EMYoga gave her an accurate and specific language to communicate back with the body.

EMYoga gives you permission, tools, and reasons to find a new intimacy with your body. This intimacy is based on self-respect and a deep love for and honoring of the physical form that carries you from cradle to grave. This intimacy requires you to touch, massage, hold, smooth, soothe, and care for your body in a way most people never do. It is a powerful permission to love yourself in this way, and it is deeply healing. To really learn how to love, listen to, and trust yourself is a big step on the way to health and healing. Simply doing the practices regularly will help you both find that intimacy with your body and learn to listen deeply to its cues.

How to Feel Energy

One of the most exciting things for new EMYoga students is to feel their own energy. It's one thing to talk about the concepts but quite another to get your hands into the energy fields and systems that run you. Some of the easiest and most effective ways to begin to feel your own energy are described below. They are presented in more detail in the practice section (part 2) of the book. Reading about them here will give you an idea of what you'll be feeling for during your practice.

PAIN

Most of you already feel the energy in the body called pain. Pain is stuck energy. When you do the EMYoga practices and come to a painful place, you're going to deeply massage, tap, draw figure eights over, or smooth the area. Unless that pain is caused by an injury or disease, massaging it is always helpful. Pain is the body's way of trying to get your attention. When the pain is acute, you listen right away. Many of you will find that when you start to palpate the body, there is pain in places you never touch. This is part of tuning in to the language of your body and learning to communicate with it when it whispers.

PRANA

Prana is the Sanskrit word for "life force" or "vital energy." When you feel buzzy after a yoga class, you've likely activated prana in the body. Prana is a very subtle energy, and as energy, it needs space to move. When you do long holds in yoga, the belly of the muscle relaxes, which then increases its overall blood supply and allows the pranic energy to move.[1]

Most of the energy you'll feel with EMYoga is prana, your own life force. There are different names for the kinds and sources of energy, but if you're feeling energy move in your body, you're awakening prana.

FEEL YOUR AURA

Rub your hands together and shake them off. Hold your hands about two feet apart and slowly bring your palms together. Many people feel a denseness when their hands start to approach each other, as if compressing a cloud. That denseness is the aura emanating from the hands. If you don't feel anything, try the same movement with your wrists. Potent points on both your hands and wrists emit energy, and some people are more likely to sense that energy at one or the other of these junctions.

Once you start to feel that energy between your hands, you'll have an easier time feeling it when you "weave" your aura (described in part 2) and whenever you sweep your arms up or down during poses. If you move your hands slowly through the "weaving," you can start to feel the threads of energy that surround you.

POINTS

Many of the holds in the practices focus on certain points. You'll hold points in pairs to help strengthen or calm meridian energy. You'll hold points on your head to release excess or old stored emotions. You'll hold your electric points. You'll hold chakras. Each of these holds will guide the body to a different outcome. However, the sensations you'll feel in your hands, things such as warmth, heat, and pulsations, are similar no matter what the hold is for. If you're holding two points, the pulsations will start to synchronize. The electric points may make your fingers feel almost like they're burning. All of these sensations are energy moving and expressing itself in your body.

BE PLAYFUL

Don't worry about what a pose looks like. Ask yourself, how does this pose feel? If you come at the pose from a feeling sense, you'll start to understand and reap deeper benefits. Start to feel the energy of the pose, which comes from its structure and how prana is moving through it. When in eagle pose, for example, you could spend your time deepening the bend in the legs or opening the shoulders. Or you could ask yourself, what does an eagle feel like? Eagles are not flying around struggling with balance or looking for points of focus or thinking about their feet. They are flying! Soaring. Seeing vast distances effortlessly. Draw that feeling into your body—*embody* the pose. This imprints the energy of the pose into the cells and is far more important than crossing the arms and legs exactly right and being perfectly still.

BE IN NATURE

Being out in nature is one of the best ways to feel your own energy and the energy of the earth, and to synchronize the two. A major healing tenet of both Chinese Medicine and Ayurveda—after finding balance—is a connection with the natural world. The vibration of the earth is itself healing, and walking barefoot allows this energy to flow up through energy points on the bottom of your feet, which activate all your energy systems. There is also an energy field that bathes the planet, called the Schumann Resonance, which is the frequency of calm, stability, peace, and vibrancy. When you leave the loud frequencies of a city or town, or even your own house, which is full of humming appliances, Wi-Fi interference, and EMFs (electromagnetic frequencies), you become immersed in the healing frequency of the planet. You can feel this energy in your body as a wave of peace.

ACCESS HEALING EARTH ENERGY

Sit against a tree with your bare feet on the earth as a way to ground yourself and access earth energy. It brings a deep calming to the nervous system.

VISUALIZATION

Another powerful way to feel your energy is by using visualization. If you are unable to perform the yoga asanas or are suffering from an ailment that makes movement difficult or impossible, you can still access the huge power of your own energy by visualizing the practices in your mind. Many studies have shown that visualization impacts the body the same way as actually doing a physical practice. For example, weight lifting in your mind actually increases your muscle mass.[2] Even if you don't have physical limitations, it is fun to practice in your mind and feel the energy moving without moving your body.

GROUND WITH SPOONS

Keeping yourself and your energies grounded is important both physically and psychologically. *Grounding* is one of those words that has transcended the yoga world. People talk about feeling ungrounded, which means they have a hard time being present, getting work done, or staying connected to themselves and others. And this is exactly what happens when we're ungrounded. We've got energy flying all over the place, but it's very hard to direct and use that energy for our own purposes.

A simple way to ground is to walk barefoot on the earth, but sometimes that isn't easy. Maybe you live in a high-rise or in a big city where there is lots of concrete, or maybe the ground is covered in snow. A great, easy way to ground is to take a stainless steel spoon and rub the back of it all over the bottoms of your feet. Another great thing to do with your spoon, after you wash it off, is to press the back edge of it around the inside of your mouth, pushing out your cheeks. This provides a really good stretch to the face muscles from an angle we don't generally get, and it resets all the valves in your body.

SHIFT ENERGY WITH THE FINGERS AND TOES

One easy way to work with a specific meridian that may be out of balance is simply by activating it. The intelligence of the body can often shift its own energy with a minor intervention such as waking up an energy. Each of the fingers and toes is a beginning or end point of the twelve major meridians. The meridians that begin or end on the fingers are Heart, Small Intestine, Triple Warmer, Circulation-Sex, Large Intestine, and Lung. And on the toes are Bladder, Gallbladder, Kidney 1 (bottom of the foot), Stomach, Liver, and Spleen.

By tapping, pinching, or flicking those points, you can awaken that meridian energy and often get it unstuck and flowing, which will help bring back balance. This is why we flick our fingers during some of the EMYoga practices. This is also why mudras (hand positions) are used so often in yoga. You're activating a meridian energy, which then activates its governing organs, muscles, nerves, and hormonal systems. Without needing to know the whole pathway of a meridian, you can affect it by simply tapping, flicking, or holding the end point of that meridian.

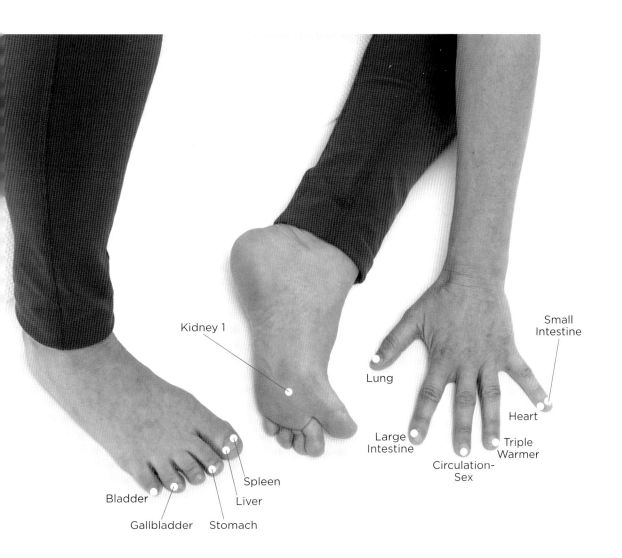

Kidney 1

Lung

Small
Intestine

Heart

Large
Intestine

Triple
Warmer

Circulation-
Sex

Spleen

Liver

Bladder

Gallbladder   Stomach

Energy Testing

One of the best tools to have at your disposal is a method for determining if what you're doing is working, if the area you're concentrating on is the right one, if the food you're choosing is beneficial, or if the supplements you're taking are correct for your body. Energy testing is this tool.

Energy testing is a way to ask your body if what you're doing is having a positive impact energetically and if it is strengthening to the body or to a particular system or making you weaker. Energy testing is both deceptively easy to do and incredibly complex and nuanced. Like diagnosing, it is both an art and a science.

Despite the learning curve and practice hours required to become a master at energy testing, it is still incredibly beneficial to tune in and start to ask the body instead of the mind (or instead of *just* the mind) the questions you have. Doing so also strengthens your intuition muscle. The more you start to listen to the cues your body is giving you, the stronger you become because the body always knows what's good for it. *The body never lies.* It always knows whether something is helping it or harming it. Therefore, you can start to see how your choices are impacting your overall energy and make your decisions accordingly.

I learned to energy test during my very first class at Innersource. The basic mechanics of it are quite simple and easy to practice. We deliberately call it "energy testing" as opposed to "muscle testing," which is from the Touch for Health and kinesiology schools, because we are testing the energy flows and how they react to certain introduced currents. We are not testing the strength of the muscle. This is particularly important when working with men, because some men tend to view muscle testing as a competition to see who is stronger. The process of energy testing becomes easier once you understand that you are simply working with an acceptable amount of force to gauge if the energy flows or not.

The best and most comprehensive directions for learning energy testing is in Donna Eden's book *Energy Medicine*.[3] If you really want to hone your skills, that is the place to go.

I'm going to give you a thumbnail direction here so you can get started.

LEARN ENERGY TESTING

The easiest way to learn energy testing is with a partner.

Stand facing your partner and ask them to hold an arm out to the side at shoulder height. Put one hand on their other shoulder and one hand on their outstretched wrist. Make sure they have an open palm, not a fist.

First, you want to get a "testable muscle." Say the person's name and have them repeat it:

You say: "My name is Sally."

They say: "My name is Sally," as you apply downward pressure on their arm and they try to resist. The arm should remain strong.

Next, you test for a "negative" to make sure the test is reliable.

You say: "My name is Nancy."

They say: "My name is Nancy," as you apply downward pressure on their arm and they try to resist.

If you're testing Sally, her arm should go weak when she says, "My name is Nancy." If she stays strong for both, or goes weak for both, you both need to do the Wake Up practice (page 78) to get the energy flowing correctly. Then do these pre-tests again.

Once you have a testable muscle, you can work with a substance, a thought, a vow, or anything that you're wanting to confirm if it's beneficial to the body.

If you're testing a substance, your partner holds it against their belly. You'll then push down firmly on their wrist. If the arm collapses, the substance is not good for the person. If the arm stays strong, either not moving or moving slightly with a bounce but staying strong, then the substance is good or neutral. You can write a vow or thought on a piece of paper and test that as well. This is a fun technique to practice with children. They start to see the energetic effects of their choices while learning about the power of energy, and they're generally very willing and nonjudgmental participants.

This is a deceptively simple technique but takes some time to become your own trusted advisor. Like any other new skill, you must practice it to become proficient.

LEARN SELF-TESTING

There are several ways you can test yourself. The one I find works best is to make a human pendulum of yourself. Stand in front of something you're testing or hold it to your body and close your eyes. Take a deep breath in and exhale completely. Allow your body to either sway forward toward the object, meaning it is beneficial, or away from the object, meaning it isn't. The trick of energy testing is its nuance. You can override it if you're not paying attention. Try to clear your mind of a desired outcome, especially when self-testing.

Self-testing is a tool that needs to be used frequently to become part of your toolkit. The value comes from learning to trust your body. The more you tune in to your own energies and let them speak to you, the more you'll be able to increase your own powers of intuition and self-trust.

Tapping: A Tool for Quickly Shifting Your Energy

I wrote about tapping in my first book, and it will be a part of my next book too. Tapping is that powerful. There is a huge movement, bestselling books, online summits, and courses all over the world on Emotional Freedom Technique tapping and the healing that can come from it. It is used for a variety of issues, both mental and physical, from weight loss to PTSD. EFT uses fourteen meridian points on the body and a simple phrase to repeat. You can find resources to explore more about it at the back of the book. Here, I'll offer my interpretation of tapping with more of an EMYoga component to it.

Tapping is important both because of its simplicity and efficacy, and also because it is an energy tool that is easy to deploy and helps resolve the problem at the level of energy instead of at the level of intellect. It is incredibly difficult to think ourselves out of our behaviors or habits, especially those that start in our unconscious, where 95 percent of our behavior originates. Tapping is one of the tools that scientist Bruce H. Lipton calls "super-learning"—ways to reprogram the hard drive of our unconscious so it more accurately reflects our conscious desires. But it is not only emotional. Tapping has a huge effect on the body's physiology as well, because the emotions and the physical body are intertwined and affect each other deeply.

It's helpful to have one fail-safe go-to tool to use when you are really bottoming out from stress, anger, fear, guilt, sadness, shame, depression, or even physical symptoms such as headaches and pain. Tapping is one of those tools that could rise to the top of your list. I know it's on mine! Tapping can be used to remove negative emotions, reduce food cravings, reduce pain, and implement positive goals. The combination of tapping and voicing very particular phrases works to free the unconscious from negative patterns, releasing emotional and physical blocks from the body and mind.

When you take stock of the voices and motivations in your head, what do they sound like? Are they helpful, encouraging, loving, and cheerleading you on to your best self? Chances are they are not.

I frequently hear from men and women who outwardly look successful that inside their own minds the voices are disparaging, angry, and downright hostile. Many of these interior voices come from our preverbal stages of development, when the brain was literally a sponge and simply took all information in at face value. Those voices take on the authoritative tone of truth and become so engrained that we often don't even know they aren't "ours," and they certainly aren't serving us. We can change, remove, and reprogram the unhelpful, disparaging, and mean voices through tapping.

What follows is a streamlined, simple approach to using this tool, taught to me by nutritionist and chiropractor Dr. Julie Schleusner, who specializes in whole body healing. It essentially comes down to tapping exclusively on the pinky-side edge of the hand (which is one of the points in the full EFT protocol). This is a Small Intestine point, which decides what is important to keep or discard both physically, and energetically. It is coupled with the Heart meridian, which informs that decision for our highest good. Tapping here aligns those energies quickly and harmoniously.

We take things a step further by homing in on the idea that almost all issues can be reduced to the two root emotions of fear or shame. You can get right to the heart of an issue when you can find the part of it you fear or are ashamed about.

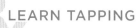

LEARN TAPPING

Find an issue that is troubling you. Start to tap on the pinky-side edge of one hand with the fingers of the other hand while saying one of the following statements aloud:

"Even though I fear [your issue], I completely love and accept myself 100 percent, 100 percent of the time."

"Even though I'm ashamed of [your issue], I completely love and accept myself 100 percent, 100 percent of the time."

You can scroll through a hundred options in your mind as you're tapping. When you get to the one that elicits a strong emotion, such as a gut punch, tears, or rage, it will immediately flood your body. This is where the "juice" is. This is where the unresolved emotion is hanging out, causing problems. This is what you'll use in the statement as you tap. And you'll tap on the pinky-side edge of the hand, using the same phrase that elicited that response, until you feel no more "charge" with the statement. Including the phrase "100 percent, 100 percent of the time" allows love and self-acceptance to penetrate even into areas you might not be aware of.

By speaking to the body in the language of the body, you override the messages and habitual patterns that have been unconsciously driving you and start to repattern and reprogram your mind and body for health.

LEARN TEMPORAL TAPPING

Another powerful tapping protocol is used to shift our habit fields, our morphic fields, as described in chapter 1. It is called the Temporal Tap. Tapping along the cranial seam on the temporal bone helps to calm the fight-flight-freeze response and is used to help shift habits. Tapping along this pathway calms Triple Warmer, the system that holds our habits. By tapping backward along this path, you momentarily stop the input of the millions of bits of information flooding your unconscious and insert a new thought "habit"—directly impacting your unconscious programming.

Loving the self is such a universal challenge due to the core paradox that we are wired to evolve beyond the self and at the same time we need to love and accept ourselves. So this is where we start. I often give the following very simple Temporal Tap practice to students, no matter their struggles.

Stand in front of a mirror and look yourself in the eye. This seems to increase the power of this practice. Bring the thumb and first two fingers of each hand together into a little "beak" and tap each "beak" firmly along both sides of your head, from the temples, around the ears, to the back of the head. Tap with a bit of firmness, and at the same time repeat the phrase "I love myself" or "I am happy" or "I am peaceful." You are tapping in an affirmation. Your phrase should feel possible, positive, and desirable. State it in the present tense, for example, "I am healthy" or "My life is full of abundance" or "I am peaceful." (See the online video for a demonstration of this technique.)

If it is difficult for you to stay positive, or countering voices rise when you're tapping in your affirmation, take your hands and smooth behind your ears on this same path. Then try it again. If it still feels difficult, you may want to try the first tapping protocol in this section to clear some of the negative voices in your head.

A way to work with this is to say three phrases. The first is something good about yourself that is absolutely true right now. If you have difficulty accepting or loving yourself, this is a great place to begin. Find a positive quality about yourself, even if it's something small, such as "I like my hair" or "I'm a nice person" or "I cleaned the whole house today." Then add two phrases that you'd *like* to be true, such as "I am completely healthy" and "I love myself." Use the three together so that you start with a statement you fully accept and then begin to program your unconscious to bring about the conditions described by the second and third statements.

Repeat the phrases and the tap at least three to five times while looking at yourself in the mirror. Do this practice every day for a month. A good time to use this ultra-short practice is right before you step on your yoga mat for your full EMYoga practice. Be alert for even miniscule improvements and describe them in your journal. You reinforce what you recognize.

3

The Five Elements

I n order to bring things in balance, it is helpful to have an energy system that speaks to all of the other systems. The Five Elements is that system. It speaks to our body's energies in relationship to each other and is both a map to identify where there may be imbalances and a tool to balance them out. It speaks to the emotions, our psychology, and the physical body, helping us see and heal ourselves holistically. It uses sound to reach into the organ systems and works directly with emotions—the often overlooked link to disease.

From the ancient Chinese term *wuxing* ("five processes" or "five phases"), the Five Elements theory is one of the major systems of thought within Chinese Medicine. From Dondi Dahlin's wonderful book *The Five Elements*, we get the most comprehensive idea of what this ancient system is: "In *The Inner Canon*, a 2,000-year-old medical text, Chinese physicians and scholars theorized that the universe is composed of forces that include water, wood, fire, earth, and metal—the Five Elements. They proposed that human behavior, emotions, and health are influenced by these elements and that people's personalities could be distinguished by them."[1]

Also thought of as phases, the Five Elements are "the underlying energy patterns that flow through and leave their imprint on all of the other energy systems . . . They provide a lens for understanding and working with chronic health issues, behavioral patterns, and emotional challenges."[2]

Each element aligns with a season and emotions, governs two to four meridians, and rules parts of the body. Together they can help you see yourself as part of a much larger system, a drop of water in a vast ocean. In a complex world, they give you a way to understand yourself in relation to the enormous workings of the universe, of which you are a part.

This chapter will explain the power of the Five Elements system, your emotions (which they govern), and all the ailments they can heal by bringing them into balance. In the next section, you'll learn the individual physical practices.

Which Element Are You?

Each element has certain characteristics associated with personality traits, body types, and emotional and health tendencies. Every person has a primary and secondary element. Once you know what your primary element is, it can help you understand not only your psychological predilections but also your potential pitfalls or weaknesses. Knowing your element helps you understand how you are in the world and gives you insight into how to manage your world so you can remain balanced and healthy. Also, knowing the element that is least represented in you gives clues to what you may need more of to come into balance.

Your primary element is the filter through which you see and interact with the world and your relationships. If all is in balance, you might not see your main element, but you tend to get ill and get well through that element. It doesn't so much define you as interpret you. It gives you some guiding principles to help you understand how you operate physically and emotionally.

The following short quiz will help you determine your primary and secondary element (as well as your least-represented element). When answering the questions, try not to think about them too much. Go with your gut. Answer the questions based on your current reality rather than what you wish to be true. The element with the highest score is your primary element, and the element with the second highest score is your secondary element (and obviously the one with the lowest score is your least-represented element). If two elements tie, they will be your primary and secondary elements.

The Five Elements Self-Inventory

Rate each of the statements below on a scale of 0 to 5, where 0 is never true and 5 is always true. Then tally your scores for each element.

WATER	SCORE
I yearn for meaning for my experience on earth.	
I am suspect of people and their secrets, and I do not want my secrets exposed.	
I am very introspective, can pull deep into myself, and can cut off from the world.	
Ideas, more than people, stir my soul.	
Fear is the emotion that disables me the most.	
I tend to believe that the world is a dangerous place and that one needs to be careful.	
It takes me a while to really trust someone.	

WOOD	SCORE
I am very assertive and clear about where I stand.	
I can marshal my intellect, and my vision can lead others.	
I am bold and decisive.	
I am fiercely independent.	
I enjoy organizing and structuring any situation.	
I get muscle tightness or tension.	
When someone is obviously being treated unfairly, I stand up for the oppressed.	

FIRE	SCORE
Feeling panic is very familiar.	
I am spontaneous, optimistic, and energetic.	
I am a very passionate person.	
I laugh and/or giggle a lot.	
I often get tongue-tied or mix up my words.	
I love safe, heartfelt contact with others.	
If my close relationships are not stable, I am not stable.	

EARTH	SCORE
I find myself in the middle a lot.	
I am naturally compassionate and supportive.	
I love spending time with my family and am the hub of family or social networks.	
Everyone confides their secrets and stories to me.	
I would never humiliate anyone publicly.	
Activities such as cooking, music making, gardening, homemaking, sewing, woodworking, and crafts are very important to me.	
I have some problems in balancing the needs of others with my own.	

METAL	SCORE
I tend to be neat and orderly in my personal surroundings.	
I put virtue and principles before fun.	
I like tasks that require systematic, logical, and analytic problem solving.	
Integrity and excellence are extremely important to me.	
I hunger for what seems to be an unattainable spiritual connection.	
I take pride in being efficient and methodical.	
I appreciate it if I can do more and be better than others.	

SCORES

___   ___   ___   ___   ___

How Emotions Affect Your Health

The Five Elements system gives us a simple and unique way to understand and work directly with our emotions. Dr. Candace B. Pert, the brilliant, groundbreaking neuroscientist, was the first person to prove that our brain chemistry is affected by our emotions. But she went a powerful step further when she proved that it's a two-way street: not only is our brain chemistry affected by our emotions, but our emotions are affected by our brain chemistry.[3] The problem is, we rarely learn how to deal with our emotions. They tend to get a bad rap in our modern world, from our reliance on diagnostic tests and computers for telling us what's wrong with us to the hyperdramatic emotionality of reality TV. But emotions serve an important purpose in guiding us, and now, with this newer brain chemistry understanding, in healing us.

Emotional intelligence didn't come into vogue until the late 1980s through the work of John Mayer and Peter Salovey. It was then further expanded with Daniel Goleman's book *Emotional Intelligence*, published in 1995. Finally, we were given tools and a deeper understanding of how our unprocessed emotions affect us.

Many of us learned to ignore our emotions, stuff them down with food or other addictive substances, or be victims of them, swinging wildly from emotion to emotion with little understanding or ability to integrate what they were trying to tell us.

In the worst instances, unprocessed emotions manifest in behavior that is destructive or self-destructive. We need to be able to deal with our emotions when they come up. We also need to deal with the emotional issues that occurred in the past and are lodged in the body, affecting us in ways we may not even be aware of. In yoga, you'll often hear the phrase "The issues are in the tissues." This speaks to the fact that if emotions aren't dealt with when they occur, they get stuffed into the physical body. Many people have been in yoga classes when an emotional release takes place. This happens because a physical area of the body where an emotion is stored opens up, causing an emotional release at the same time. This can be cathartic but also scary if you don't have tools for processing what's happening. Emotions are necessary and instructive. They are part of our survival mechanism, giving us instant feedback to experiences around us.

Along with working on and releasing old emotional patterns and energy held in the body's tissues, EMYoga works directly with emotions as they arise.

This is, in fact, the crux of the Five Element Flow practice (part of the Essential EMYoga practice), which is presented in chapter 4. It teaches us how to deal with emotions continuously so that they don't wreak havoc with our systems. This not only helps with mental calm, but it also helps heal physical illnesses, as the emotions are often the psychological expression of the physical symptom. Emotions are powerful cues for the body and are not to be dismissed. They are great teachers and guides to what is working and what is not working in our lives. We need to learn to harvest the information that our emotions are trying to show us and then release the energy of the emotions.

Dr. Pert articulates the power of suppressing and releasing emotions in *Molecules of Emotion*:

> Emotions are what unite the mind and the body. Anger, fear,
> and sadness, the so-called negative emotions, are as healthy
> as peace, courage, and joy. To repress these emotions and not
> let them flow freely is to set up a dis-integrity in the system,
> causing it to act at cross-purposes rather than as a unified whole.
> The stress this creates, which takes the form of blockages and
> insufficient flow of peptide signals to maintain function at the
> cellular level, is what sets up the weakened conditions that can
> lead to disease.[4]

As you practice the Five Element Flow, you will begin to see the cycles of your emotions as elemental and changeable. This helps you detach from the story of your emotions, enabling you to release them more quickly. Just as a huge snowstorm can disrupt your life for a few hours or even days but doesn't change the trajectory of your life, so you'll see your emotions for what they are, storms of feeling that pass quickly. Perhaps the "emotional storm" will require a snow day to process and understand, but then the energy should pass through. You shouldn't still be dealing with a pile of snow in August. And likewise, you needn't hold on to a difficult emotion, no matter how profound, if you have the tools to harvest its information and let the feeling go.

The Theory of the Five Elements

The theory of the Five Elements is that our bodies and our world have developed from the same star stuff: the elements we find around us. These elements form an intricate dance of give and take, movement and stillness, balance and imbalance. They feed each other and together govern all the biological and emotional systems of the body. This theory is based on natural cycles and relationships in the environment and within ourselves. It teaches us again about deep listening, paying attention, and tuning in. We start to watch the seasons with more attention: noticing the leaves budding out in the spring and changing color in the fall; watching patterns of animal traffic in the snow, the shifting of the winds. When we tune in and listen and watch the outside world, we feel awe. Connected. Gratitude. Oneness. This is the feeling of love, an awareness of the spirit or energy that moves through all things. This can happen anytime, but we have to tune in to it, and the more we do, the more it happens. When we tune in to the world around us, we also naturally tune in to the world within us. We start to listen to our own breath, hear our own heartbeat, notice when things aren't quite right, and feel awe and gratitude for the magnificence that is the human body.

The elements imply movement and process, not a fixed event. This is the reality of energy, and indeed of life. In *Between Heaven and Earth*, Harriet Beinfield and Efrem Korngold, two renowned Chinese Medicine teachers, write: "In the Chinese model, life is about the dynamic, constantly shifting relationships of one functional system with another, always within the context of the whole system. No aspects of the personality or body function as independent, discrete entities."[5] Nothing is ever just one thing; everything is interrelated.

The yogic tenet "As above, so below" finds its roots in Chinese philosophy. "Patterns in nature are recapitulated at every level of organization—from the rotation of the planets to the behavior of our internal organs. These ancient Oriental ideas conform to what some modern thinkers call the 'holographic paradigm': the organization of the whole (nature) is reflected by each and every part (plants, animals, human beings)."[6] This idea is congruent with Rupert Sheldrake's morphic fields, capturing the idea of resonant habits at every level of organization in a system. This is not just a metaphor or New Age idea. There is actually a scientific, mathematical expression of organic structures in nature called fractals, which appear from a repeated equation. You can learn more about fractals from stem cell biologist Bruce H. Lipton,[7] but in essence the equation shows us that the formation of an eye is similar to a solar storm; our blood pathways are similar to a river or the branches of a tree. It helps us see ourselves in the patterns of the universe. It proves the adage "As above, so below," so we stop seeing that as a hopeful metaphor and start to see it as the truth of existence. This helps us understand why working with the subtle energy can have such profound effects to the physical body. If you change something at one level, it must shift on all levels. As above, so below.

The Five Element Wheel

The Five Elements system is depicted as a wheel with a five-pointed star in the middle, connecting the elements in two different patterns. There's a circle on the outside (the flow cycle) and a star on the inside (the control cycle). This visual description helps us see how the elements (and all their constituent parts) are in a constant dance with each other.

One of the most powerful things about the Five Element Wheel is that the wheel itself can be a predictor of where we have issues in a particular element. The easiest and most holistic way to learn the Five Element Wheel is to super-impose it on your own body. This is how we learn to use the wheel in diagnosis and treatment at Innersource. It makes sense that the body would offer a simple way to both diagnose and heal itself. After all, we existed for thousands of years without the technological diagnostic tools used today. The body has its own built-in, easy-to-use system to understand what's wrong with it, and to help get it back on the right path.

The pattern of the Five Element Wheel on the belly is the physical identifier for an element out of balance. This check-in, called the Starfish Connection (see the online video), will help you see where energy may be stuck. Daily palpate this wheel to discover where there is soreness (or if you energy test, you can discover where energy weakens).

You'll start palpating on the lower right, in water, which governs teeth, bones, and all bodily fluids except blood. This area is located in the lower right of the abdomen, near the hip bone. It is approximately over the bladder. Press in with strong pressure, massaging deeper than the surface muscle layer. When massaging the flow wheel, you'll be massaging in the direction that digestion happens

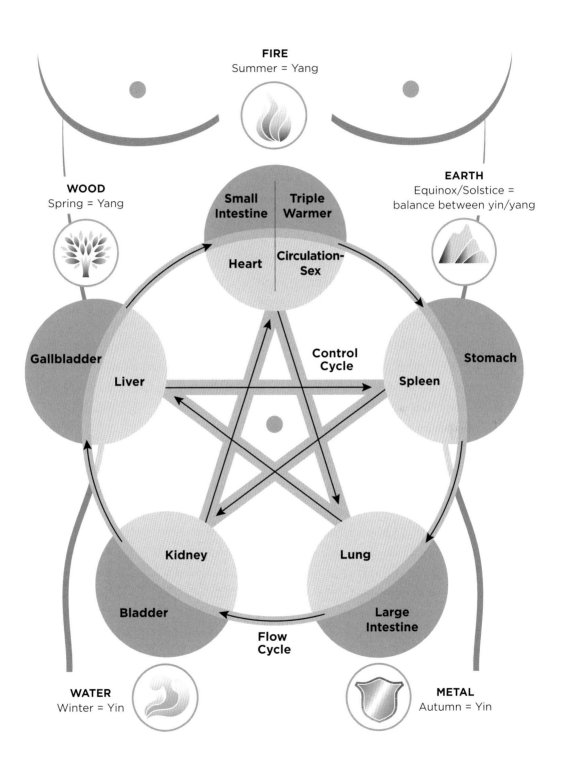

FIRE
Summer = Yang

WOOD
Spring = Yang

EARTH
Equinox/Solstice =
balance between yin/yang

Small
Intestine

Triple
Warmer

Heart

Circulation-
Sex

Gallbladder

Liver

Control
Cycle

Spleen

Stomach

Kidney

Lung

Bladder

Large
Intestine

Flow
Cycle

WATER
Winter = Yin

METAL
Autumn = Yin

in the body. This in itself is a great way to help your digestion. You need to digest your emotions as well as your food to maintain health. If when you palpate this area it is sore, it can indicate something is out of balance in the water element. The main challenging emotion is fear, balanced by courage.

Move on to wood, which governs muscles, tendons, and ligaments. The main challenging emotion is anger, balanced by assertiveness. It is located in the upper right, just out from the bottom rib over the largest part of the liver. If it is sore when you palpate this area, it can indicate something is out of balance in the wood element.

Wood moves on to fire. Fire is located at the xiphoid process, where the rib cage meets in the center at the bottom of the sternum. It points toward the ruling organs of fire: heart and pericardium. Fire governs blood vessels. The main challenging emotion is anxiety, balanced by inspiration or joy. If the area is sore when you palpate it, this can indicate something is out of balance in the fire element.

Fire moves into earth. Earth governs blood. The main challenging emotion is overcompassion for others, balanced by compassion for the self, self-love. This area is located on the left side of the upper abdomen, approximately where the stomach and spleen lie. If this area is sore when palpated, it can indicate something is out of balance in earth.

Earth flows into metal. Metal governs skin and hair. The main challenging emotion is grief, balanced by letting go. This area is in the lower left of the abdomen, near the left hip bone. It lies over the large intestine. If when palpated it is sore, it can indicate something is out of balance in metal.

After you massage the flow cycle, massage the control cycle, pressing your fingers in with some pressure starting at the lower right (water), up toward the xiphoid process (fire), down to the lower left (metal), up to the upper right (wood), then to the upper left (earth), and back down to the lower right (water). This gives you information about where energy may be stuck on the control cycle, moving from one element to the next. This is also a way to quickly clear energy. If you do the Starfish Connection daily, you start to see where there is work to be done. If there is any pain and it doesn't resolve easily, it may be pointing to something larger at play within that element.

You can also understand yourself and your energy challenges by studying the markers of personality and archetype. The Five Elements help us understand how our personalities are geared toward a specific tendency. If you're a wood element, you tend toward anger as your default out-of-balance emotion. If you're a water element, you likely get caught up in fear. The goal is to get off the "wheel" of difficult emotions—to stop being reactionary to situations, flung around by emotionality. I suggest reading Dondi Dahlin's book for deeper source material about the Five Elements in your personality.

In the same way that the elements work with the cycles of the seasons, they work with the cycles of our emotions. Our emotions transition in a similar way. Fear often transmutes into anger and then into anxiety. From there we can go into a self-lacerating reaction where we forget ourselves and start to care too much about everyone else in a situation, and then we move into grief. It is a familiar and repeatable challenge.

One of the biggest hurdles to overcome is our own resistance to feeling emotions. Emotions can be scary or painful or uncomfortable. We feel ashamed or afraid, and we don't want to feel that way. Or we see how we are punishing someone by being emotionally distant or cruel, and then we have to look more deeply at our own behavior and feel compassion for ourselves, even when we aren't at our best. We avoid our feelings so much that they literally cause us to become sick. In order to deeply heal, we have to be willing to step into the fear of our own feelings and let that feeling release itself as raw energy—that is the scary part. We fear that the rage, grief, or anger will last forever and we will never get away from it. But the truth is, emotion is just energy, and when we remove the story, the energy will run down in a finite amount of time. Once the raw energy of the emotion releases, it's gone. It's when we don't release the emotion that it continues to fuel the difficult and detrimental story it hatched from and then can often become a physical illness.

The beauty of the Five Elements is that they show us cycles within cycles. Everything runs in cycles—the day, the week, the month, the year. Our bodies have different cycles of eating, sleeping, activities, and cleansing. Every experience cycles through the elements. In a day, we wake up in the watery realm of quantum possibility, move into the wood of movement, into the fire of getting things done, then the warmth of nurturing yourself and family at the end of the day, and finally we move into metal, reviewing and releasing the day and going to sleep.

The Five Elements system helps us understand our personalities, physical tendencies, and ways of getting sick and healing in the world. Just as the seasons go round and round, so our life and our patterns turn. This is important to remember when we're going through a difficult time—nothing stays the same; our lives are in constant transformation. By using this system as a lens to see ourselves, we get a broader, more comprehensive view of our whole being. This gives us a distinct advantage when trying to figure out the pieces that need healing in our lives.

USE THE ELEMENTS TO BALANCE THE ELEMENTS

You can help balance your elements with external tools. If you're working with fire, bring some literal fire into your life. Light candles, build a small bonfire in the backyard, and write down things you want to give up as well as bring in to your life and offer them to the flames. If you need more metal, consider wearing some metal jewelry, or like me, take a welding class. You can use the actual elements themselves to bring physical balance. Plant a garden (earth), take a steam sauna, go sit by a river or ocean (water), or get some of the deliciously smelling Paulo Santo (wood). When your element is out of balance, you can use the elements themselves to help bring you back to peace.

Sound and the Five Elements

Sound is a key part of working with the elements, as every element has its own healing sound. This gives us a precise and direct entry to working with both the conscious and unconscious effects of emotion.

Sound is so powerful in transforming energy because in reality, at our most basic level, we are all simply vibration. By changing our vibration, entraining our fields to a more coherent, organized frequency and literally "tuning" our bodies, we can affect the largest change with the least amount of effort.

The "brains" of cells are the skin or the membranes of the cell, and these membranes hold little antennae that cause them to be exquisitely sensitive to sound and vibration. They react and interact with our entire body and the world around us by picking up and reading the surrounding frequencies.

With our own breath and vocal cords, we can create coherence in our body, leading to balance and healing. In fact, the vagus nerve (extending from the brain stem to the abdomen) has been shown to promote healing and happiness, and is activated by singing and humming. The hyoid bone, the only bone in the body that is not connected to any other bone but is free-floating, is located in the throat, behind the voice box, and vibrates and moves as you sing and hum and speak. Attached to nothing (similar to the idea of nonattachment in yoga), it helps us find, through our voice, our truth.

In this book, we'll use the main sounds of the body's organs, as determined by Chinese Medicine, to help balance and heal their corresponding systems. We'll use these sounds within each element practice. But you can also use them on their own, whenever you feel the need to release excess emotion.

USE THE FIVE ELEMENTS SOUNDS TO HELP RELEASE EMOTION

The sounds of the five elements are:

Water: *whoooo*

Wood: *shhhhh*

Fire: *haaaaa*

Earth: the sound of ujjayi breath (described in chapter 4)

Metal: *ssssss*

YIN-YANG THEORY

The yin-yang theory is the theory of opposites. We are constantly moving between magnetic poles. The search for balance is the movement between these two poles. The idea is to bring opposites together, not to join but to continue the dance. Yang is the masculine, active, outward-moving force. The yang points start or end on the head and travel down the back of the body. Yin is the feminine, receptive, inward-moving force. The yin points start or end on the core and run up the front of the body. The symbol of yin-yang holds that the polar opposite still exists in the extremity of its opposition. In EMYoga, we bring this awareness of duality and create bridges between those opposites. Balancing our own masculine and feminine forces—our physical oppositions as well as our mental oppositions—are all part of the practice. Bringing the body into dynamic movement with great stillness holds the power of what is called the coexistence of opposites. Holding both stillness and movement at the same time increases our power. Stretching the body wide and drawing it in small expresses this idea in physical form.

Each element holds two meridians (except fire, which holds four), a yin and a yang meridian. So within each element there is a masculine external force and a feminine internal force. For example, the yin of water is like a deep interior well or spring; the yang expression of water is like a bursting geyser. That applies to the emotions as well. Out-of-balance yin in water would be fear turned inward: maybe you're afraid of your own life, making the wrong choices, not being enough. A yang imbalance would be fear of the outer world, events, or circumstances. This can help you determine if you need to have a quieter yin practice (to calm the yang) or a more active yang practice (to counter the stillness of yin).

The yin-yang theory is also the start of movement. A juggler starts with one ball and tosses it back and forth between her hands. This is yin-yang: back and forth. When you add a second ball and then a third, you start to throw them up and across each other and catch them with opposite hands. This is the star inside the wheel—the control cycle. This is dynamic movement. When you get really good, you can toss the balls around in a circle—the flow cycle. Back and forth (yin-yang) then grows to the dynamic interplay of many moving objects in a constant dance (the Five Elements).

There are many ways to use the information in this book, whether you're completely healthy and thriving in your life and yoga practice, or if you're struggling with issues physically, emotionally, or mentally. I encourage you to adopt a playful attitude, no matter the circumstances of your life. You can go through this book sequentially, or just flip it open and see what jumps out at you. You can do the practices exactly as written or adapt them based on other techniques you already use or knowledge you have.

The most important thing to remember is the key to your own health and happiness is in your own hands. Yes, we often need help, but at the root of it all, your own body holds within it everything you need. This is one of the basic tenets of yoga, and it follows here with Energy Medicine Yoga even more.

Once you start to work with these simple tools, you'll see your own abilities and health increase dramatically. Even if things in your life seem challenging right now, if you enter this work with a sense of curiosity, you'll be rewarded more than you know.

TABLE 1 Five Elements Body Ailments

	water	wood	fire	earth	metal
abdomen, swollen				x	
abdominal muscles, weak	x				
abdominal pain			x	x	
acne	x				x
adrenal exhaustion			x		
allergies		x	x	x	x
anemia				x	
angina			x		
ankles, swollen and weak	x				
appetite, excess				x	
appetite, loss of	x				
armpit pain or swelling			x		
arms/legs, heaviness in				x	
arteries/blood problems			x		
arteries, hardening of the	x				
arthritis	x	x		x	
asthma			x		x
awkward movements					x
back pain, low	x				x
back tightness, upper		x			
beer belly			x		
bloated				x	
blood pressure, high	x	x			
blood pressure, low	x		x		
blood pressure, unstable		x			
blood problems				x	
blood sugar disturbances				x	
blushing			x		
body temperature, low				x	
body tingling, twitching, or numbness		x			
bone problems	x				
bowel disturbances					x
breast problems				x	
breast soreness			x		
bronchitis					x

	water	wood	fire	earth	metal
bruise easily				x	
bursitis	x				
calf pain	x				
cancer of all kinds		x			
candida		x			
capillaries, broken				x	
carpal tunnel syndrome			x	x	
chest congestion					x
chest pain			x		
chest tightness		x			
chills			x		
chills and heats easily			x		
chronic fatigue syndrome	x				
circulation, poor					x
circulation problems			x		
colds					x
colic					x
complexion, flushed or pale/ashen			x		
congestive heart failure					x
constipation					x
coughs					x
craving sugar or caffeine				x	
cysts, lumps, growths		x		x	
dermatitis, contact					x
diabetes			x	x	
diarrhea					x
digestive problems		x	x	x	
dizziness		x	x		
ear problems	x		x		
ears, ringing in		x	x		
eating disorder				x	
eczema/psoriasis					x
edema	x			x	
elbow problems	x				
emotional shock			x		

TABLE 1 FIVE ELEMENTS **BODY** AILMENTS (CONT.)

	water	wood	fire	earth	metal
energy/stamina, lack of	x			x	
erratic pulse			x		
exhaustion			x		
eye diseases		x			
eye pain		x			
eyes, bags under				x	
eyes, dark circles under	x				
eyes, itchy		x			
fainting spells			x		
fallopian tube issues				x	
feet, flat, and fallen arches	x				
feet, sweating	x				
fever			x	x	
fibroid tumors				x	
flu					x
fungus		x			
gallstones		x			
glands, swollen			x		
gluteus, sore			x		
grinding teeth		x			
gum disease					x
gums, bleeding or swollen			x	x	
gums, weakening	x				
hair loss, balding, premature gray	x				
hair, brittle or dry	x				
hands/feet, cold	x				
head, heaviness in				x	
headaches	x	x		x	x
headaches (forehead/frontal/occipital)	x				
headaches, dull				x	
headaches, one-sided		x			
headaches, temple		x			
hearing deterioration	x				
heart disorders	x		x		
heartbeat, irregular/rapid			x		

	water	wood	fire	earth	metal
heartburn				x	
hemorrhoids				x	x
hepatitis		x			
herpes/cold sores					x
hip problems		x			x
hives			x		
hormonal problems			x		
hot flashes			x		
hunger, frequent				x	
hypersensitivity to light and noise	x				
hypertension		x			
hypoglycemia			x		
immune deficiency syndrome	x			x	
immune function, depleted					x
impotence	x		x		
infections				x	
infertility	x				
insomnia			x		x
intestinal/colon disorders				x	x
jaundice		x			
jaw pain		x			
joint pain	x				
joints, brittle	x				
joints, weak				x	
kidney stones	x				
knee problems	x	x	x		
laryngitis				x	
legs, weak			x		
lethargy		x			
libido, low	x				
lightheadedness			x		
limbs/joints, achy				x	
loose stools				x	
lymph swelling				x	
menopause issues		x	x		

TABLE 1 FIVE ELEMENTS **BODY** AILMENTS (CONT.)

	water	wood	fire	earth	metal
menstrual flow, heavy				x	
menstrual irregularities	x	x			
metabolic disorders				x	
migratory pain		x			
mineral deficiencies					x
moles/warts					x
mood swings			x		
morning fatigue			x		
mouth, bitter		x			
mouth sores			x	x	
mucus, thick				x	
muscle tone, poor				x	
muscles, stiff/tight					x
muscles, weak				x	
muscular tension/cramps/spasms		x			
nails, cracked/dry/soft					x
nails, hard/cracked		x			
nasal polyps					x
neck pain or tension	x	x		x	
nerve problems, trigeminal			x		
nervous system problems	x				
nervous tension				x	
nervousness		x			
neurological disturbances	x				
nipple pain			x		
nose problems					x
nose/throat, dry	x				
nose/throat/sinuses, congested					x
obesity				x	
osteoporosis	x				
ovarian problems	x			x	
palpitations			x		
periods, irregular		x			
perspiration, excessive			x		
perspiration, lack of	x				x

	water	wood	fire	earth	metal
pleurisy					x
PMS		x	x	x	
pneumonia					x
posture, stiff					x
pregnancy problems				x	
prostate problems	x		x		
respiratory symptoms					x
sacrum problems			x		
saliva, excess or lack of				x	
sciatica	x	x	x		
scoliosis	x				
sedative abuse		x			
sensitivity to climate changes					x
sensitivity to smells					x
sexual problems	x		x		
shallow breathing	x		x		
shingles		x			
shortness of breath					x
shoulder pain		x			
sinus problems				x	x
skin/lips/hair/nails/nasal passages, dry					x
skin, oily, or acne		x			
skin, prematurely wrinkled	x				
skin problems					x
skin rashes, hives, eczema, or other irritations			x		
sleep disturbances	x	x	x		
slow at healing cuts				x	
sneezing or coughing bouts					x
speech disturbances			x		
sperm count, low		x			
spine, inflexible					x
spine/joint problems					x
spine, weak/stiff	x				
stimulant abuse		x			
stomach, acid imbalance in				x	

TABLE 1   FIVE ELEMENTS **BODY** AILMENTS (CONT.)

	water	wood	fire	earth	metal
stomach/intestine/bladder/uterus, prolapsed				x	
strain injuries		x			
swallowing difficulties				x	
tendon injuries		x			
thigh circulation and strength, lack of			x		
thighs, achy				x	
thirst, excessive	x				
throat problems	x				
throat, sore				x	
thyroid, hyper or hypo			x		
thyroid problems	x			x	
tinnitus			x		
TMJ		x			
toenails, thick		x			
toes, pigeon	x				
tongue, red/inflamed			x		
tooth decay				x	
tooth/gum problems	x				
tooth loss	x				
toothaches					x
toxicity		x			
tuberculosis					x
ulcers				x	
urethra/anus, itchy		x			
urinary or bladder problems	x				
vaginal infections	x				
varicose veins	x			x	
vertigo	x				
vision deterioration	x				
vision, blurry		x			
visual disturbances		x			
weight problems			x	x	
yeast infections	x				

Adapted with permission from Innersource Class 5 handout.

TABLE 2 **Five Elements Mind Ailments**

	water	wood	fire	earth	metal
absentmindedness	x				
addictive relationship with food				x	
aggression		x			
agitation and irritability		x	x		
ambivalent and wishy-washy				x	
antisocial tendencies	x				
anxiety, general feelings of		x			
apathy	x				
aversion to cold/winter	x				
blocked creative energy		x			
burnout			x		
caught in the middle				x	
clinging relationships				x	
compassionate to a fault				x	
compulsive need to help				x	
constant need to be needed or included				x	
craving for sweets and carbohydrates				x	
cut off from others	x				
cynicism	x				
deep feelings of impotence and frustration	x				
dependency on external stimulants and sedatives		x			
depression	x				
depression (with anger)		x			
difficulty getting started on projects				x	
difficulty in conflict and disorder					x
difficulty letting go of the familiar					x
difficulty paying attention and thinking logically due to lack of energy and vitality			x		

TABLE 2   FIVE ELEMENTS **MIND** AILMENTS (CONT.)

	water	wood	fire	earth	metal
difficulty relaxing		x			
difficulty separating thoughts from feelings			x		
difficulty with changes and transitions				x	
disorganization			x		
eagerness to please			x		
easy to judge others					x
emotionally inaccessible	x				
emotionally unstable			x		
emphasis on order					x
emptiness				x	
excessive concern for the feelings of others				x	
excessive criticism	x				
excessive desire for cold drinks			x		
excessive giggling and laughter			x		
exhaustion			x		
extreme anxiety			x		
fanaticism	x				
fear of being confined or controlled by others		x			
fear of being disconnected or homeless				x	
fear of failure					x
fear of inability to ignite others			x		
fear of losing control					x
fear of ridicule		x			
feelings of abandonment				x	
feelings of being stuck or trapped		x			
feelings of helplessness or hopelessness		x			
feelings of inadequacy				x	
feelings of loss of control				x	
feelings of shame, embarrassment, or humiliation		x			

	water	wood	fire	earth	metal
flat and mechanical emotional responses					x
flightiness				x	
forgetfulness			x		
formal/stuffy presence					x
forsaking themselves				x	
free-floating anxiety			x		
frustration		x			
gloomy/cheerless demeanor	x				
haughty and aloof personality					x
hypersensitivity to criticism				x	x
hypochondriac tendencies	x				
hysteria/delirium			x		
inability to adapt to change					x
inability to concentrate or pay attention			x		
inability to move forward with ideas and plans	x				
inappropriate loud or annoying laughter			x		
indecisive behavior		x			
inflexibility	x	x			
insecurity	x				
insensitivity to other's feelings/needs		x			
intense need to be accepted			x		
intolerant of opposing viewpoints					x
irrational thought patterns			x		
irritability	x				
lack of aggressiveness				x	
lack of appetite			x		
lack of confidence	x				
lack of energy				x	
lack of inspiration and creativity					x

TABLE 2 FIVE ELEMENTS **MIND** AILMENTS (CONT.)

	water	wood	fire	earth	metal
lack of interest in food	x				
lack of motivation and willpower	x				
lack of originality and creativity					x
lack of spontaneity			x		
lack of trust	x				
laziness	x				
loneliness				x	
loss of faith in self	x				
loss of passion			x		
loss of will to live	x				
meddlesome behavior				x	
monotonous, droning voice			x		
mood swings			x		
muddled or confused thought patterns			x	x	
nervousness				x	
not feeling supported while supporting others			x		
not giving to self				x	
obsession with cleanliness					x
obsessive relationships					x
obsessive thoughts about sex	x				
obsessive worrying				x	
overeagerness to please			x		
overgiving to others				x	
overly critical and judgmental					x
overpowering desire to win or accomplish a goal		x			
overwhelm			x		
overwhelming need to stay in touch with others				x	
panic			x		
paranoid tendencies	x				
pessimism	x				
phobias	x			x	x

	water	wood	fire	earth	metal
poor judgment in love issues			x		
preoccupation with own thoughts and low interest in others	x				
procrastination	x				
questioning of authority		x			
rapid speech pattern			x		
restless/nervous energy		x	x		
ritualized routines					x
self-centeredness	x				
self-destructive behaviors		x			
self-righteousness					x
skeptical, aggressive tendencies		x			
sluggishness				x	
smoldering anger turned inward		x			
strict disciplinarian					x
sudden and irrational outbursts			x		
suspicion of others	x				
tendency to be critical of others					x
tendency to be overly serious		x			
tendency to be petty and judgmental					x
tendency to be unforgiving	x				
tendency to blame others		x			
tendency to blame self		x			
tendency to equate love with loyalty	x				
tendency to go off in several directions at once			x		
tendency to make life difficult for others		x			
tendency to wallow in past grief					x
tendency to wear heart on sleeve			x		
tendency to withdraw and isolate when stressed	x				
tendency toward prejudice					x

TABLE 2 FIVE ELEMENTS **MIND** AILMENTS (CONT.)

	water	wood	fire	earth	metal
unexplained fears	x				
unexplained or chronic sadness					x
unfocused goals/directions	x				
unfocused or scattered thought process				x	
violent outbursts of anger		x			
withdrawal from others		x			
workaholic		x			

Adapted with permission from Innersource Class 5 handout.

To access videos
of the following
practices, please visit
soundstrue.com/emyoga

PART 2

Body

The Energy Medicine Yoga Practices

Physicians talk about breakthroughs in personalized medicine and pharmacogenetics—using information from a person's genetic map to tailor medicine to his or her own particular needs. But yoga can already do that. It can turn our bodies into customized pharmaceutical plants that churn out tailored hormones and nerve impulses that heal, cure, raise moods, lower cholesterol, induce sleep, and do a million other things. Moreover, yoga can do it at an extremely low cost with little or no risk of side effects. It has the potential to usher in a genuine new age.

WILLIAM J. BROAD
The Science of Yoga

4

Foundation Practices and the Essential Energy Medicine Yoga Practice

The Essential EMYoga practice is what I consider the foundational practice to keep yourself healthy, your energies humming along, and everything working well. If this practice is new to you, I suggest doing it daily for a month so you can start to see some real, direct results. This will also bring you a familiarity with some of the poses that may seem strange at first. Once you feel comfortable with it, you can move on to the individual element practices as needed.

Every EMYoga practice includes a focus on breath, meditation, and the use of bandhas. These techniques are explained in this chapter.

Pranayama: Breathing Practice

No matter which practice in this book you are doing, the breath is an integral part of it. Your breath is the direct link between your mind and body and is one of the most powerful tools in yoga. Your breath patterns give a view into the emotional disturbances in your body, and by working directly with your breath, you have the opportunity to clear these. The breath is also a link between the conscious and the unconscious mind. To unite the mind and body in health, you need to unite the often opposing ideas of the conscious and unconscious mind. Our breath holds one of those important keys. When you intentionally control your breath and guide it into certain patterns, you affect the habitual patterns that are held in your energy fields. If you are habitually hurried, nervous, anxious, or scared, for example, you can affect the habits of those feelings by consciously breathing in a way that calms those habits down.

There are many wonderful books that discuss pranayama in depth, but here I briefly outline the basics. Each of the Five Element EMYoga practices in this book has its own pranayama, either at the start or at the end. As a general rule, practice five minutes a day (up to twenty) of pranayama by itself. To get started, try this:

1 Massage the Lung neurolymphatic points (shown on page 195).

2 Massage the first point on the Lung meridian.

3 Free the diaphragm (shown on page 196).

4 Place a drop or two of essential oil on the inside of the wrist crease. Bring your wrists to your nose and deeply inhale while cupping your fingers around your eye sockets, then open your hands out and cup your fingers around your ears. (The inner wrists hold points for Lung, Heart, and Circulation-Sex meridians, which bring the plant wisdom of the essential oil you choose directly to that organ.) Now begin the breathing practice of your choice.

FRANKINCENSE: MY NUMBER ONE ESSENTIAL

Although the study of aromatherapy and essential oils is a huge one, I like to simplify things. I generally carry three to five essential oils with me when I travel, but if I had to choose only one oil to have with me at all times it would hands-down be frankincense. The pure, therapeutic-grade oil has many uses, including as an antimicrobial and antibacterial. It is good for balancing hormones, creating healthy mouth bacteria, digestive issues, wrinkles, and skin care, as well as eliminating resistant cancer cells and protecting against radiation (which is why I use it while flying or getting X-rays). And it smells wonderful! You can put a drop or two on the inside of your wrists before you do your pranayama practice.

Ujjayi: Victorious Breath

Ujjayi is the breath used most often in yoga classes. It increases physical power by pressurizing and directing the breath. It is heating and a means of dissipating and controlling pain. You will do this breath throughout most of your EMYoga practice.

You can learn the ujjayi breath with your mouth open or closed, but it is generally practiced in yoga classes with the mouth closed. To try it, slightly constrict the glottis at the back of your throat, forming a whispering sound on both the inhale and exhale. Some people call this the Darth Vader breath because of how it sounds. Your breath should be audible to you, but not so loud that someone across the room can hear it. If you're having difficulty getting the hang of it, put your hand in front of your mouth and exhale a breath as if you're fogging a window or a pair of glasses. Then try the fogging exhale again, this time with your mouth closed. Again, you should hear the fogging Darth Vader sound on both the inhale and exhale.

YOGA BREATH VERSUS ENERGY MEDICINE YOGA BREATH

In most yoga classes, the instructions are to breathe in and out through the nose. This type of breathing helps contain and build energy. It is also a form of biofeedback that shows you where you are in your yoga practice; if the physical work gets too challenging, the breath rate increases, and you may feel the need to open your mouth to let more oxygen in. But breathing through your mouth incites a stress response, the exact opposite of what you're hoping to achieve with yoga. So instead of defaulting to a mouth breath to meet the physical demands, you should slow down the physical practice. As you get stronger in your practice and build lung capacity, you are able to work harder physically while still maintaining a nose-breathing pattern.

In EMYoga, there are times when you breathe in through your nose and out through your mouth. This breathing helps facilitate and reinforce the connection between the Central and Governing meridians—the core energies on the trunk of the body. They connect where the hard and soft palates meet at the top, back of the mouth. Try taking one breath and pay close attention: inhale through your nose and exhale through your mouth. You can feel a circle with your breath. You feel your breath coming in your nose, and when you exhale through your mouth, you physically feel your breath at the top of your mouth. The in-breath touches the out-breath there. This type of breathing is also used in the Taoist meditation known as the microcosmic orbit, a technique for cycling energy through the body.

Another important reason to exhale through the mouth is that it releases excess energy. During an EMYoga practice (or any yoga practice, for that matter), as you move stuck energy, you may feel overwhelmed by emotion. A way to facilitate the release of that emotion from the body is to exhale through the mouth.

As you spend more time in your EMYoga practice, you'll start to build the knowledge and intelligence needed to know when a mouth exhale is necessary or when to slow down the physical work to maintain a nose breath.

For the Wake Up, the opening sequence of techniques in any EMYoga practice, you'll breathe in through your nose and out through your mouth. As you move on, you'll adopt the yogic breath of in the nose, out the nose. Tune in to your practice and watch your breath. It will become one of your greatest teachers.

Meditation

Each element practice has a meditation at the end, focusing on the practice you just completed. The meditation allows you to feel, experience, and tune in to what just occurred energetically in the body. This is another time of "stillness," where you harvest the benefits of the practice. This is the time of integration energetically. It is an important and delicious part of the practice; please don't skip it.

Bandhas

These are physical "locks" in the body, places where you can hold and direct energy to increase power and the detoxifying effects of the practice. They are both energetic and physical locations that give you an entry into moving energy. They are crucial, as they help to support the energy in the core of the body. Having access and working knowledge of the bandhas is one of the keys to longevity. There are three of them. (For more detailed directions on accessing the bandhas, see *The Heart of Yoga* by T. K. V. Desikachar.) I suggest spending some time focused on learning the bandhas and steadily building them into your yoga practice, developing your understanding of them as you go. Studying with a teacher who can assist you with the bandhas is also a great way to learn them.

Mula bandha   Located at the floor of the perineum, at the base of the body, mula bandha is activated by engaging the muscles used to stop excretions from the body. Used in standing, balancing, and seated poses, this bandha will help you stabilize and strengthen your practice. Once you learn to engage those muscles, you must learn to release them as well. Practice pulsing this bandha in connection with the exhaled breath. Start in a pranayama practice, and move with it to the asana practice when you feel ready.

Uddiyana bandha   Located between the navel and the lowest rib, this bandha helps support the core of the body. It is accessed on an exhaled breath by drawing the belly button in and up toward the spine. It helps to stabilize and energize the core.

Jalandhara bandha   Located at the throat, the jalandhara bandha helps contain the energy in the core of the body so it doesn't rise and exit from the crown. It also helps the stability and lengthening of the spine. It is activated by a slight downward movement of the chin toward the chest. It is best used in standing poses and lying-down poses.

Take Your Time

The Essential EMYoga practice takes about thirty minutes. You can add on time for a breathing and meditation practice. Each of the element practices is between an hour and an hour and a half, the length of an average yoga class.

If you're healthy now, then the time you devote daily to your EMYoga practice can vary from thirty minutes (a very good baseline) to an hour and a half or two hours. It's better to practice every day for thirty minutes than once a week for two hours. So maybe you practice thirty minutes a day, and then do a longer practice once or twice a week and take one day completely off. If, however, you are working with a health challenge, you really need to put the time into shifting your energies to bring you back into balance and full health. You'll have to gauge the time given to your practice based on your own abilities as well, especially if you're suffering from something that saps your energy. At the very least, spend the time each day to get yourself out of homolateral movement (when the body's energies are running in parallel lines) into a crossover pattern. That is the root cause of every dis-ease, and it takes little time, but frequent application, to get those energies to cross over and stay crossed over. (The Wake Up on page 78 will teach you this.)

If something is out of whack in your system, chances are pretty high that the Triple Warmer system is complicit. That may seem strange because Triple Warmer is supposed to be the energy that keeps you alive—after all, it governs your immune system. But that's just it. It keeps you alive. It isn't concerned with you transforming, even into better health. Triple Warmer can hold on tight to how you are in the moment, even if how you are is unwell. Working with Triple Warmer to relax its grip allows you to come back into a balanced and centered place. And working with Triple Warmer can take time. Triple Warmer doesn't just shift immediately. It has spent years, decades even, holding on tight to keep you alive, and it isn't going to just let go because all of a sudden you're aware of its existence. Doing things such as the Triple Warmer/Heart mudra and the Triple Warmer/Spleen hug, as well as sedating Triple Warmer and activating Radiant Circuits (all explained in part 2) help your body relax its hypervigilance so you can move into a more evolved healing place. Triple Warmer is in the fire element, and many of its calming techniques can be found there.

Selecting a Practice

Regardless of your current health status, coming into balance is the main goal. If you are sick or struggling with a health issue, it is more obvious that your underlying energy systems are out of balance, since this is what precipitates illness. To achieve and maintain health means processing your emotions as they occur and dealing with physical cues of trouble as they come in whispering, instead of waiting for them to come in screaming.

The Essential EMYoga practice (described below) is a complete routine that helps organize, balance, and clear all of the energy systems in your body, as well as provide the physical stretching, releasing, and opening you've come to expect from yoga. It is a great baseline to do daily. It introduces you to the main energetic concepts in your body and starts the "conversation" and your ability to communicate in the language of your body: energy.

There are also five elemental healing practices, one for each element. Here are some ways to use these practices:

- **Learn EMYoga with a friend or two.** Read one of the practices out loud to a friend or group. Reading the instructions starts the body's energies moving right away by letting you visualize the practice in your mind. Practicing EMYoga with friends is a great way to increase learning and to build community.

- **Work with a health challenge.** Look up your ailment in the tables (pages 52–64) and do the associated element practice.

- **Work with your health history.** Go through the ailment tables (pages 52–64) and check off the ones you currently have or have suffered from in the past. Focus on the element practice with the most entries.

- **Stay in balance.** Do the Essential EMYoga practice. Then do each of the element practices in order.

- **Work seasonally.** Focus on the element practice for the season you're in or about to enter.

- **Work with an emotion.** Choose the element practice that governs an emotion that is challenging you.

- **Work with your own element.** Choose the practice of your primary element (to discover your primary element, see the quiz on page 39).

- **Work with the emotions altogether.** Do the Essential EMYoga practice with a deeper focus on the Five Element Flow.

The role of the body's energy systems in maintaining health and well-being cannot be underestimated. Nor can the incredible changes that can happen with even a slight intervention. In *Energy Medicine*, James L. Oschman, writes: "The helmsman can change the course of a huge vessel virtually effortlessly by applying a small adjustment to the tiller. Likewise, a small energy field applied at the appropriate place and time can shift the course of an organism."[1]

The Essential EMYoga Practice

The Essential EMYoga practice is the quickest way to get all the energy systems of the body awake and moving in the right direction. (See the online video of the entire Essential EMYoga practice.) It takes about thirty minutes to do, depending on how long you spend resting in savasana. It can serve as your daily practice, and you can make it longer by adding in bits of the Five Element practices too. The Essential EMYoga practice not only activates and organizes all energy systems of the body, but it also clears toxins out of the organ systems.

The following list explains the energy of the practices presented in the pages to come.

- The Wake Up literally wakes up the body's energies and gets them moving forward and crossing over, the two most important directions of energy in the body. *This is the single most important technique in the book, and if you do nothing else, Do This Daily!*

- By smoothing, palpating, and holding certain areas of the body, you activate and guide these energy systems to do their work efficiently, easily, and joyfully.

- The squat and hang poses work with the denseness of the physical form, helping to open it up, allowing for the expression of contraction and expansion.

- The yin-yang flow smooths all the meridians in their optimum directions: yins upward, yangs downward.

- The Five Element Flow helps move energy through the emotions, releasing and processing both old and new emotions. It also shows you where work still needs to be done. If doing one of the poses elicits a powerful response, you might go to that particular element and work with it on a deeper level.

- The bridge pose helps clear toxins; doing an inversion increases the release of those toxins out of the body.

- Working the Electrics activates the electrical component of each energy system.

- Clearing the chakra channels at the throat clears all the chakras; if there is soreness, that tells you where you need to focus more work—which chakra energy is holding or triggering you at the moment. Linking the chakras after that helps soothe and bring more communication within the body.

A note on points: There are many points on the body you'll use in EMYoga. The points for working with meridians are very tiny. You'll cover these points in the meridian holds with two or more fingers, sometimes your whole hand. There are hundreds of meridian points on the body, and it's impossible and unnecessary to learn them all. When they appear in the practice, the points are noted in parenthesis after the instructions of how to hold them. This is for referencing if you'd like to know the exact location (yinyanghouse.com can help you find the exact locations). You don't need to remember the numbers of any of the points; they are there for reference and are shown directly on the body on photos in some instances to help you modify the practice. You can hold the points in many different poses and ways. If a particular pose isn't accessible to you, simply find one that works with your body, holding the points in another way.

The Essential EMYoga Practice

1 Wake Up

The Wake Up has four parts: the four thumps, the cross crawl, the zip up, and the hook up.

The Four Thumps

Thump (by pressing your first two fingers and thumb together into a little "beak" or making a fist) on point Kidney 27, then thump the other points shown. Thumping these points wakes up your energies and gets them moving forward, jump-starts your immune system, helps integrate and digest your experiences and substances, and grounds you.

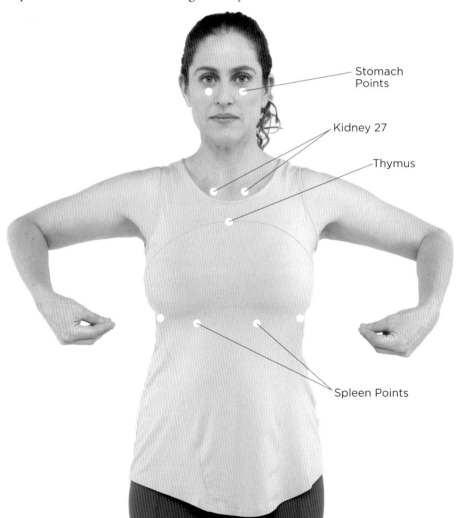

Stomach Points

Kidney 27

Thymus

Spleen Points

Cross Crawl

March in place, striking your right knee with your right hand as your knee rises, your left hand striking your left knee. After ten to twelve of these, brush your hands together as if dusting them off. Now do twelve crossover marches in place with each hand slapping your opposite knee. Your right hand slaps your left knee; your left hand slaps your right knee. If you find the crossover march challenging, it is quite likely that you need to do it more.

If you are physically unable to do the cross crawl standing, you can do it sitting in a chair, moving just your arms and not lifting your legs and knees at all. You can also visualize the practice and get your energies moving by moving your attention.

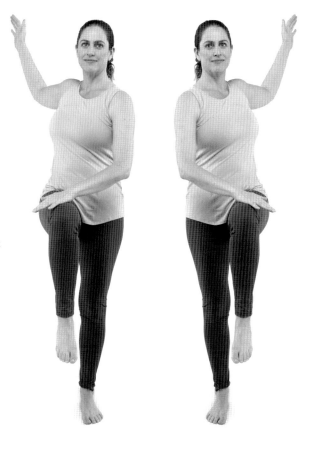

Zip Up

Hold your hands in front of your pubic bone, palms facing your body, and run your hands up the front of your body to the level of your chin. Your hands can be either touching your body or just off your body an inch or two. The movement is similar to swiping the screen on a smartphone or tablet device.

Tip: You can use this motion to seal in an affirmation for yourself or set an intention at the beginning of your EMYoga practice. Simply pause with your hands at your pubic bone, take a moment to connect to your affirmation or intention for the practice, and then zip up the words along with the energy.

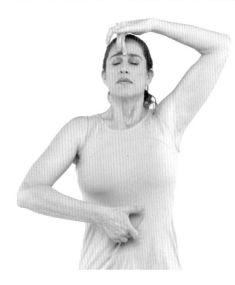

Hook Up

Put one finger in your belly button and one finger at your third eye, between your eyebrows. Push both in gently and pull slightly up. Take three deep breaths, inhaling through your nose, and exhaling through your mouth.

2 Celtic Weave to Full Forward Bend: Clear the Gates

Uttanasana

Weave your arms back and forth in front of you as you come over into a full forward bend. While bending forward, clear the gates of your hands: massage down between the long bones of your hands and pinch off in the gullies between your fingers. Then massage down your fingers themselves and pinch the tip of each finger. If you encounter any pain or soreness, spend a bit more time massaging those points. Next, do the same thing for the gates of your toes. Massage down between the long bones on your feet, pinch off in the gullies between your toes, and then pinch the tip of each toe.

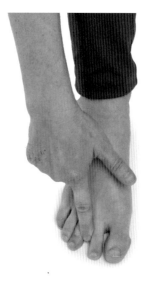
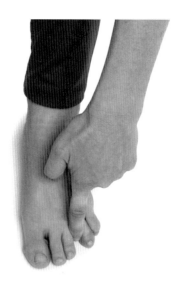

3 Squat with Twist

Come down into a squat with padding under your heels if they don't reach the floor. Bring your right arm between your legs, rest your palm on the floor, and lift your left arm up, coming into a twist. Circle your left wrist several times. When you're ready to release, smooth your left hand back and forth, through your aura, in a figure eight pattern until you bring your arm between your legs and twist to the other side.

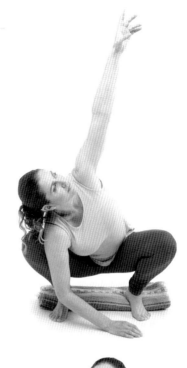

4 Hang with Spleen Trace Up
Uttanasana

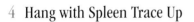

Come back into a full forward bend and then slowly come up, tracing the path of the Spleen meridian with the palms of your hands. Vigorously massage the end points of the Spleen meridian.

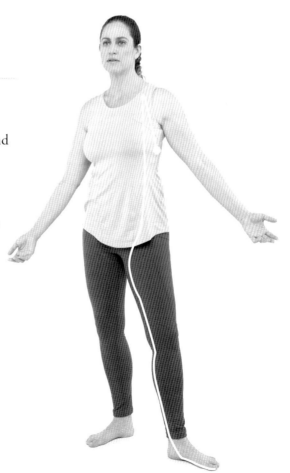

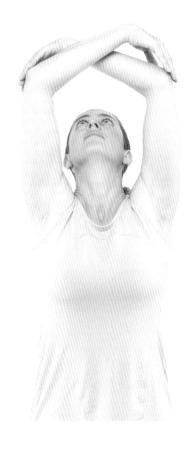

5 Yin-Yang Meridian Clear

Sweep your arms up overhead. Cross your right hand over the outside top of your left and start to smooth down the back of your left arm. At your elbow, both hands continue to smooth down the backs of your arms. Continue to "hug" across at your shoulders and down your upper back at your shoulder blades (you can bring your hands off your body into your aura if you need). You'll need to let go of your body and bring your crossed "hug" to your waist. At your waist, draw your hands apart over your belly so they're now open at your waist. Smooth your hands down the outside of your body, down the outsides of your legs, and off your pinky toes. Rise up tracing the Spleen meridian. Repeat starting with your other hand on top. Don't rise up after the second clear, but stay in full forward bend and continue to the next asana.

6 Lunge

Step your left foot back and release your left knee to the floor. Sweep your right arm open to the side, and then circle your right arm backward three times in line with your body. Stop when your arm is extended toward the ceiling and flick each finger against the thumb to activate the meridians. (Don't switch sides yet; flow into the next five poses.)

7 Extended Side Angle

Parsvakonasana

Lift your left knee off the floor, turn your left heel toward your body, and stand on your foot, rotating your body to the left. Come into an extended side angle pose with your right elbow on your right knee. Circle your left arm back as if you are spinning a pizza, arm parallel to the ceiling, not in line with your body. After three full circles, keep your arm open and flick each of your fingers against the thumb, then all of them together. Weave your arm back and forth as you bring your body forward and come onto your hands and knees.

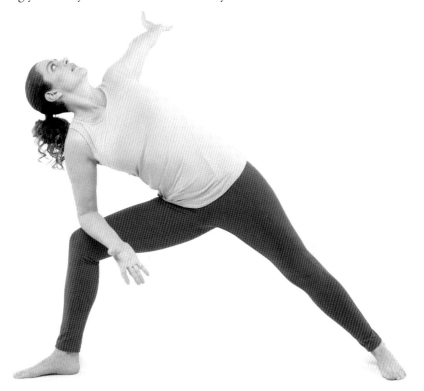

8 Cat-Cow

Inhale and lift your spine into an arch. Exhale and sink your spine into a hammock. Do this several times. Take a few breaths to arch your spine side to side as well, making your body into a crescent moon shape.

9 All Fours to Child's Pose

Balasana

Release into child's pose (see page 114) on an exhale. Inhale and come back onto hands and knees. Exhale into child's pose. Do this five times.

10 Downward Dog to Upward Dog

Adho Mukha Svanasana to Urdvha Mukha Svanasana

Come into downward dog and take five full breaths. Inhale and come forward to upward dog. Exhale and come back to downward dog. Move between downward and upward dog five times. Use mula bandha strongly to protect your low back. Alternately, you can move from downward dog to plank and back to downward dog.

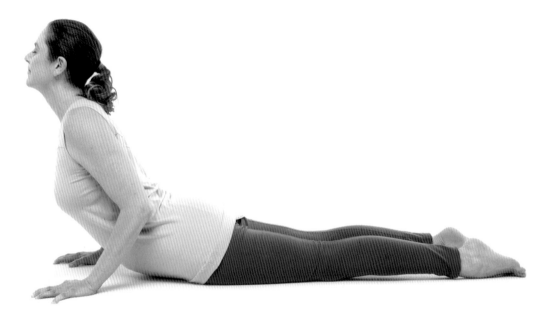

11 Triple Warmer Rock

From upward dog or plank, slowly lower your hips and then your upper body to the floor as if you're coming down from cobra (see directions on page 118). Stack your hands one on top of the other and rest your forehead on your hands. Rock your hips side to side on the floor. Press back to downward dog and repeat the sequence (poses 6 through 11) on the other side, stepping your left foot forward between your hands and letting your right knee come to the floor for a lunge. After the final downward dog, walk your feet back toward your hands and hang over in a full forward bend for a few breaths.

12   Hang with Arms Overhead

Uttanasana

Interlace your hands behind your body and then lift them overhead, stretching your shoulder girdle. Stay here several breaths.

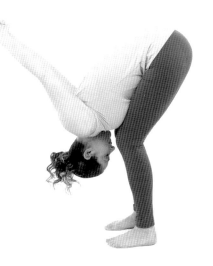

13   Chair with Penetrating Flow

Utkatasana

Bend your knees, sinking into chair pose (utkatasana). Bring your arms to your low back. With your hands together, massage your low back around and around in a big circle. Keep circling your low back as you lift your trunk up while keeping your legs bent in chair. Rise to standing and flatten your hands on your low back, then smooth them around to your groin. Flip your hands back and forth several times in front of the junction of your groin and your upper thigh. Smooth your hands up over the front of your body, over your chest, and cup your hands around your mouth. Make three audible exhales, then come to stand with your hands over your heart.

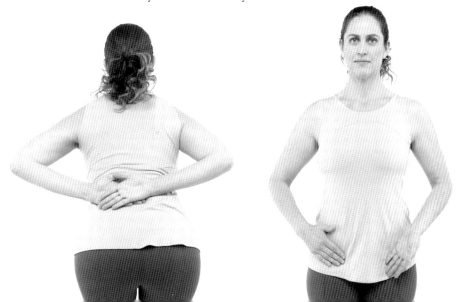

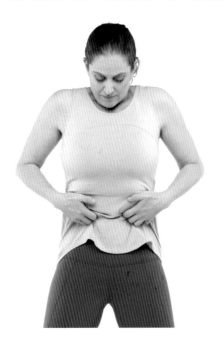

14 Ileocecal/Houston Valve Clear

Stand with your feet slightly more than hip-width apart. Bring your hands flat over your low belly, with your pinky fingers on the crest of your hips. Inhale and press your fingers deeply into your belly and pull upward. Exhale and shake off your hands. Bring your hands to the same position and do it again. Inhale, pressing deeply in and pulling up. Do it one more time. Now bring your hands to your low ribs, inhale, and on your exhale, press your fingers deeply in and smooth down. Shake off your hands.

15 Five Element Flow

Each of the following five poses is the peak pose for one of the elements. Doing them one after the other helps move the energy of the corresponding element's emotion out of your body. Feel free to do this whole sequence two or three times.

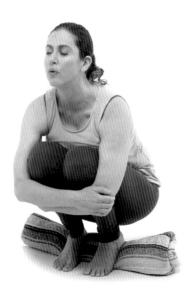

Blowing Out the Candle (*Water*)

Squat with a rolled-up blanket or mat under your heels. Make sure your heels are anchored on the blanket. (If your heels reach the floor easily in a squat, you don't need the blanket.) Hug your arms around your knees. Inhale, bowing your head down. Look up and exhale with the sound *whoooo*. Do this three times. You can think about something you're afraid of and visualize yourself blowing out a candle, affirming that you have the courage to be in the dark or the unknown.

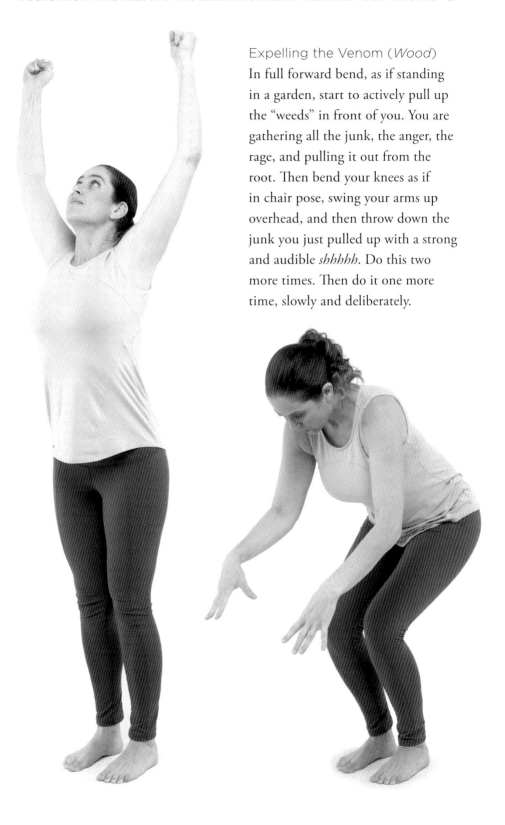

Expelling the Venom (*Wood*)

In full forward bend, as if standing in a garden, start to actively pull up the "weeds" in front of you. You are gathering all the junk, the anger, the rage, and pulling it out from the root. Then bend your knees as if in chair pose, swing your arms up overhead, and then throw down the junk you just pulled up with a strong and audible *shhhhh*. Do this two more times. Then do it one more time, slowly and deliberately.

Bringing Down the Flame (*Fire*)

Begin standing. Inhale and sweep your hands up overhead, and when they meet overhead, tent your hands together so all your fingers and thumbs are touching. Exhale with a *haaaaa* sound and bring your thumbs to the top of your head, the center of the crown chakra. Release your hands from the crown and sweep them out and around again on an inhale. Exhale with the sound *haaaaa* and bring your tented hands together with your thumbs touching between your eyebrows at your third eye.

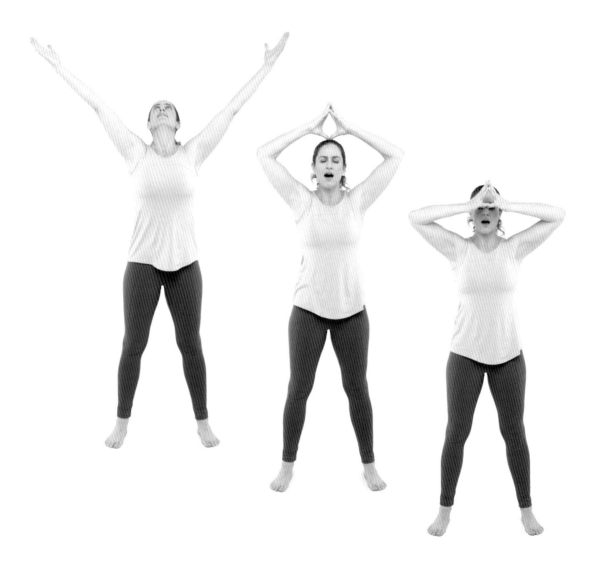

Release your hands and inhale, sweeping them around in a circle. Tent your hands, exhale *haaaaa,* and bring your thumbs to your heart center. Inhale, sweep your arms around again, tent your hands and bring your thumbs to your navel. Exhale *haaaaa.* This is where the fire wants to be seated, in your navel center. Keep your thumbs here as you inhale and bring your pinky fingers to rest on your pubic bone. Exhale *haaaaa* and flatten your hands onto your low belly, keeping your index fingers and thumbs connected.

Inhale and smooth your hands down your legs, then down and off your feet, shaking them off in front of you. Exhale with the *haaaaa* sound, and rise up while tracing the Spleen meridian. Massage the Spleen meridian points at the side body in line with the bottom of your chest. In these poses, you are reeducating the information from your fields into the wisdom of the chakra centers.

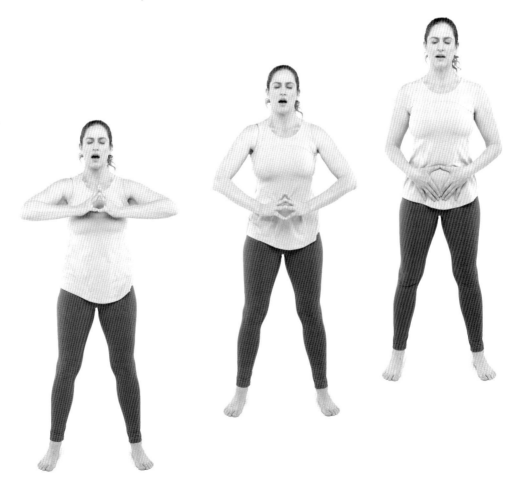

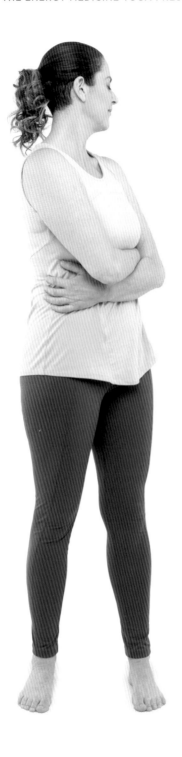

Cradling the Baby (*Earth*)

Using a strong ujjayi breath, wrap your arms around your body, giving yourself a big hug. Rock your body side to side while you're hugging yourself. When you feel complete with that, inhale and sweep your arms up overhead. Hold your breath in and pull down four times from the heavens. Exhale, sweeping your arms out and down, and come all the way forward to a standing forward bend (uttanasana). Put your hands under your feet. Inhale and pull up and away from your body; exhale and sink back down (padahastasana). Do this two more times, then finally release your hands and slowly come up, tracing the Spleen meridian. This pose feeds self-love into the nervous system.

Human Touching Divine (*Metal*)

Inhale and take a slight backbend, opening your arms with palms facing up at the level of your hips. Exhale with a *sssss* sound and bring your hands rounded together in front of you with your fingers almost, but not quite, touching. Inhale again and take a slightly higher backbend, your arms opening up around the level of your chest. Exhale with a *sssss* sound and bring your fingertips close in front of you but not touching. Inhale again, this time taking a full backbend with your arms either shoulder height or above your head. Exhale with the *sssss* sound, bringing your hands together and allowing them to touch and cross over, smoothing down your arms and over your shoulders. Stand here with your hands flattened over your chest as you inhale and exhale the *sssss* sound several times. This pose holds and releases our life experiences, teaching us about the pulse of life and that ultimately we are not in charge. To surrender fully allows us to maintain our strength.

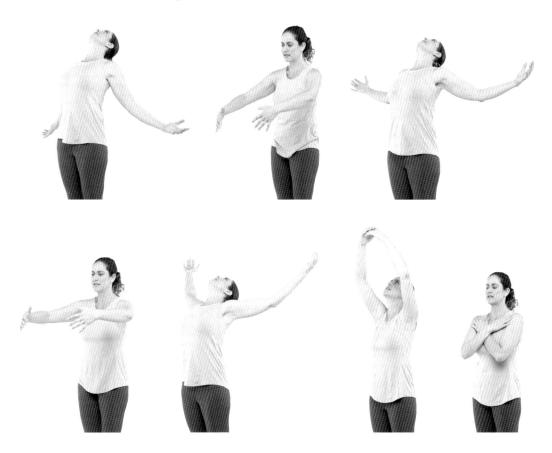

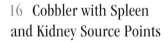

16 Cobbler with Spleen and Kidney Source Points

Baddha Konasana

From standing, slowly lower down to seated. Bring the soles of your feet together, knees out to the sides. Lean forward from your hips and bring your thumbs into the upward-facing exposure of your Achilles tendons, your fingertips to the edge of the balls of your feet. Hold for several breaths, up to a minute.

17 Slow Sit-Ups with Hook Up

Lie on your back with your knees bent, feet on the floor, hip-width apart. The farther away your feet are from your body, the easier the sit-ups are, so adjust accordingly. If doing the sit-ups with bent knees is still too challenging, you can extend your legs straight on the floor.

Wrap your arms around your torso in the Triple Warmer/Spleen hug: right hand on your left rib cage, left hand holding just above the bend in your right elbow, on the outside of your arm. You can alternate which arm is over and which arm is under. Apply jalandhara bandha, tucking your chin in toward your throat. This helps take the weight of your head off your neck and keeps you from using your neck muscles. If you feel any strain in your neck, you can do these sit-ups with your head in your hands, being sure to soften your neck completely. You are using your stomach muscles and core strength, so be mindful.

Slowly lift your body toward your bent knees. Do not use any momentum—that is the key to this posture. Go slow, slow, slow, using the deep core muscles. Press your belly down into the floor as you lift your body up toward your thighs and apply mula bandha. Come down with the same incredibly slow speed, making the muscles work on the down as much as the up. Think about pushing down to lift up. If you get to a point where you cannot lift any farther without your feet popping up, stay just before that point and keep pressing your stomach muscles toward the floor and drawing mula bandha up. Don't rock yourself up by pulling on your arms or cheating your feet off the floor. When you need to release, slowly lower down at the same speed. Do a total of three to five slow sit-ups. Then lie back and bring one finger into your belly button and place one finger at your third eye. Push both in and pull slightly up. Take three breaths, inhaling through your nose, and exhaling through your mouth.

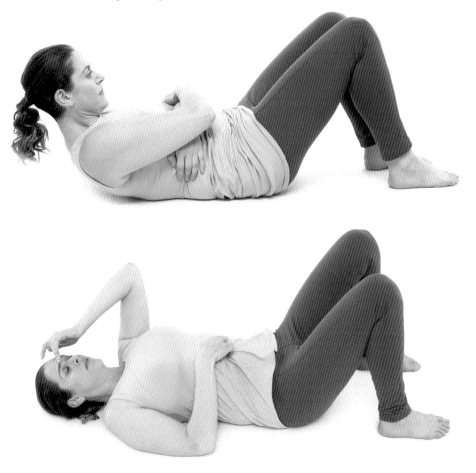

18 Moving Bridge with Neurolymphatic Point Clear for All Elements

Dwi Pada Pitham

Lie on your back with your feet on the floor, knees up. Have your feet a foot or so from your buttocks. Inhale, raise your hips off the floor, and lift your arms up until they are resting on the floor behind you overhead. Exhale, release your hips back to the floor at the same time as your arms. Repeat this five times. Inhale, hips up, arms up, exhale, hips down, arms down. After the fifth time, keep your hips up, but allow your arms to return to the floor. Continue breathing smoothly and slowly.

See if you can release your buttocks and let the work of the pose move to your feet, your low back, your shoulders, and your core muscles. Hold five breaths, and then slowly relax back to the floor. Let your knees soften toward each other. *Tip:* If you have low back issues, go back and forth between squeezing the butt muscles and releasing them. This will help strengthen your back and protect it at the same time.

While resting from bridge pose, clear all of the points shown on the facing page by massaging them deeply. Then lift up again into bridge for a few breaths. Lower down and continue.

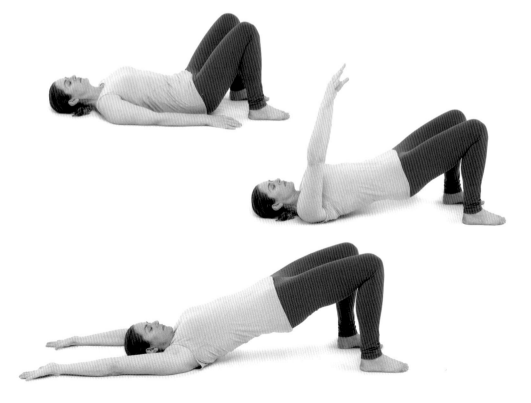

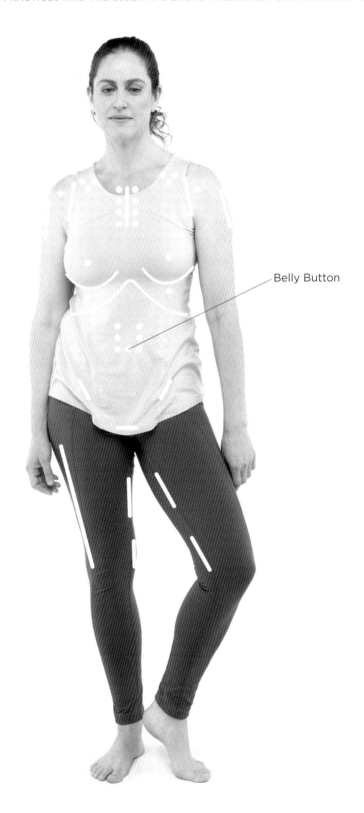

Belly Button

19 Starfish Connection

Using the fingertips of one or both hands, massage your belly in a circle, starting from your lower right and moving around in a clockwise direction. Then massage the star pattern, also starting from the lower right. (See page 44 for more details.)

20 Supported Shoulder Stand or Legs Up the Wall with Electrics

Sarvangasana or Viparita Karani

Either bring a block under your sacrum and lift your legs straight up into the air (modified sarvangasana), or bring your butt to the edge of the wall and roll onto your back, lengthening your legs up the wall with or without a block under your sacrum (viparita karani). Legs up the wall is less muscular work and more restorative. Ask your body what it needs at this point in the practice. Bring your hands behind your head. Massage deeply all along the occipital ridge, the bone at the base of your skull. You may notice several sore spots. Massage these. Remain lying down, and bring your thumbs or your first two fingers into the main electric points. These are located in the two deep hollows on either side of the ropy tendons at the back of your neck where your neck meets your skull. Allow your elbows to relax down to the floor, or use padding under them so you don't have to hold up your arms. Rest here for two to ten minutes.

You will start to feel warmth, heat, tingling, pulsations, electrical impulses, or vibrations under your fingertips. This is the electrical component of all your energy systems waking up and synchronizing. Don't remove your fingers, even if they feel funny or hot. When you're ready to come out of the pose, first, push your fingers in more deeply and massage them around, and then slide your hands outward, around, and down your neck. Shake off your hands. Slowly lower your feet, remove the block, and let your body rest here. If you're against the wall, roll onto your side and rest here.

21 Hug Knees

Still lying on your back, hug knees in and wrap your arms around them to release your back.

22 Fish with Chakra Clear

Matsyasana

Straighten your legs and let your body rest on the floor for a moment. Hug your arms into your side body, then slide your hands under your buttocks or thighs, depending on your body, and slowly start to lift your heart center up, letting the crown of your head release back to the floor. Weight is on your elbows, buttocks, and if you lower your head all the way down, the crown of your head. Stay here three to five breaths.

To release, put weight more on your elbows and lift your head off the floor, slowly rolling back down along your spine. Now with two fingers from each hand, start at the center of your throat on the Adam's apple and smooth

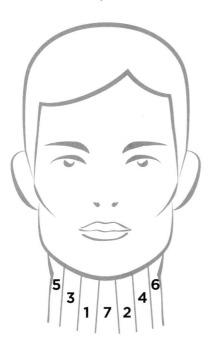

in opposite directions on an imaginary line. This corresponds to your seventh chakra and follows your windpipe. (See diagram for correspondences between the throat channels and the chakras.) Move one inch to the left and smooth the fingers up and down another "column." Continue with two more columns until you are almost to your ear. Then clear the three columns on the right side the same way, smoothing your fingers apart along the imaginary line of the column. Shake your hands off and lift back up into fish pose for several breaths.

23 Hug Knees

Again, hug knees in and wrap your arms around them to release your back. Hold for several breaths.

24 Lying Side Twist with Gallbladder Points Hold

Lie on your back with your knees bent, feet on the floor. Move your hips one inch to the left to offset your spine, and drop your knees to the right side. Let your arms come out from your body in a T. If you like, you can straighten your top leg (which will be your left). Hold directly behind your knee with your right hand. You can hold from the top or bottom; the goal is to be directly behind your knee in the popliteal crease. Breathe deeply for three to five breaths. Then gather and hug into the center, and repeat on the other side. These points, behind each knee, are called the "achievers of the impossible"—good ones to activate!

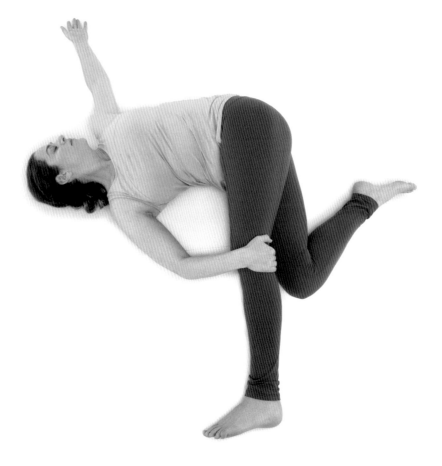

25 Savasana Prep with Chakra Link or Neurovascular Hold

Note: Choose which hold you'll do before release into full savasana.

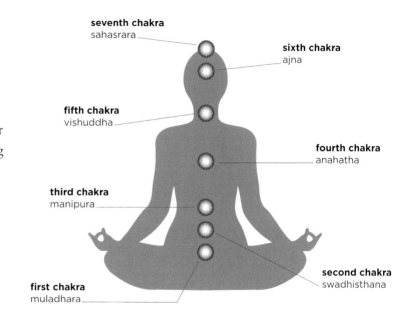

seventh chakra
sahasrara

sixth chakra
ajna

fifth chakra
vishuddha

fourth chakra
anahatha

third chakra
manipura

second chakra
swadhisthana

first chakra
muladhara

If one of the chakra channels in your throat is sore or feels like it is calling your attention, bring one hand to cover the corresponding chakra on your body. Bring the other hand to cover a chakra whose information or essence could help support the chakra you're working with. For example, if your channel on the throat corresponding to the third chakra feels sore, you'll put one hand over your third chakra slightly above your belly button, the place of personal power. Maybe you'd like to infuse that with love, in which case you'll put your other hand on your fourth chakra. Or maybe you'd like to infuse that chakra with an increased ability to communicate, in which case you'll put your other hand over your fifth chakra at your throat.

Hold your hands over the chakras for two to three minutes. Support your arms with props so you can relax here. You may feel warmth or buzzing.

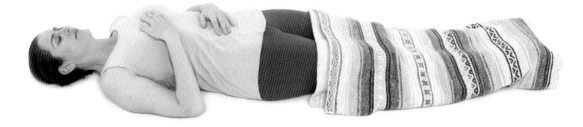

26 Neurovascular Reflex Points Hold

If you feel an emotion calling your attention more than a chakra is, do this hold before final relaxation. Place one hand on your forehead and the other on the points for the element whose energy you wish to release. See diagram for hand positions for each element. Hold here for a minute or more. Your body will tell you when it feels complete, and you can move to full savasana. If you're feeling really emotional, you can prop up your arms with bolsters and keep this hold through your entire savasana.

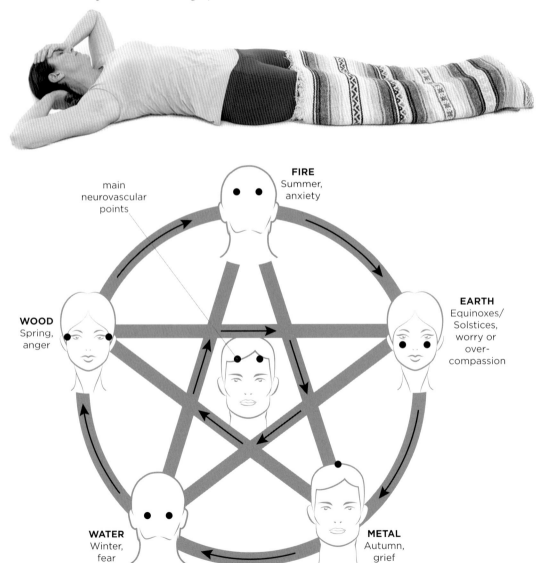

main neurovascular points

FIRE
Summer, anxiety

EARTH
Equinoxes/ Solstices, worry or over- compassion

WOOD
Spring, anger

METAL
Autumn, grief

WATER
Winter, fear

CHAKRA PERSONALITIES

Here is a quick rundown of the personalities of the chakras:

- The first chakra (muladhara) carries energies related to family, tribe, security, and sexuality.

- The second chakra (swadhisthana) carries energies of creativity, innocence, joy, and sexuality.

- The third chakra (manipura) carries energies of ego, our personal identity, and our sense of power in ourselves and in the world.

- The fourth chakra (anahatha) carries energies of love—our ability both to receive and give love.

- The fifth chakra (vishuddha) carries energies of communication and expression.

- The sixth chakra (ajna) carries energies of intuition, insight, and vision, as well as our connection to our own inner world.

- The seventh chakra (sahasrara) carries energies of our connection to the larger world and to the cosmos or the divine.

27 Savasana

Lie on your back and bring your arms down to your sides, slightly away from your body. Let your legs relax and roll open. Allow yourself to completely relax, let go, and surrender. Let the awakened energies do their work of healing and repatterning your body. This is the most important step of the practice. Stay in the pose for three to fifteen minutes.

28 Pranayama and Meditation

Spend some time doing pranayama practice (see page 69). This helps drive the energy into all your cells. Then sit in meditation for five to ten minutes, which allows your mind to absorb the practice and to pattern itself after stillness. (You can find additional instructions for pranayama and meditation practices in each of the element practices.)

ALTERNATE WAKE UP

You can do the Wake Up standing or sitting, quickly or slowly. The point is to get your body awake and to start to communicate with it. Here is an alternative you can use when you're feeling like being more still.

Stand on the bare ground. If you can be outside and barefoot, that is preferable. If you're inside, step off your mat and stand on the bare wood or bare stone. Cross your hands in front of your chest and press your fingers or thumbs into Kidney 27. Massage deeply, press the points, and then just hold your fingers here. Lean your body into your hands and press up into the points. Activate mula bandha, pressing in at the root of your body, drawing energy upward. Now hold here, pulsing both Kidney 27 and mula bandha (see the online video). Let yourself stay here as long as you need as the energy surges through your body. Once you feel awake, you can continue with the rest of the Wake Up.

5

Water

Everything starts in water. It is the womb, the realm of quantum possibilities. Corresponding with the winter season, it is the deepest, most internal time of year—the most introspective. Water is the source, the place where all is possible and from where all energy emerges. It is the imaginal realm.

In EMYoga, as in Energy Medicine, all healing cycles begin with water, and when we do an Energy Medicine session to find out where the energy is stuck, we always start with the two meridians and organ systems that correspond with water: Kidney and Bladder.

Kidney is the meridian system that leads all the others. The first acupuncture point on the Kidney meridian, Kidney 1, is the point on the base of the foot where energy enters the body. The energy then rises up to the end point of the Kidney meridian, called Kidney 27, which is a junction point for all the other meridians (located in the hollows below the tips of your collarbone). Kidney 27 (K27) is considered the "on" button of the body, and thumping or tapping or deeply massaging this point awakens all the energies of the meridians and gets the body's energy moving forward, which is one of the two most important flows of energy in the body. If the body's energy isn't moving forward, you are working at a 50 percent deficit. This means that the body can't heal itself. It is moving against its own energy. It's like rowing against the current of a river.

The Psychology of Water

In terms of psychology, the water element is the energy of the baby, the philosopher, and the king. This can be powerful, potent, and, when out of balance, dangerous. Think of a despot king who believes he is right, entitled to anything he wants, and cares little for the needs or feelings of others. The main emotion that causes problems when water is out of balance is fear. And fear (along with anger, which is the wood element) can be one of the most debilitating and dangerous of emotions.

Winter, the season associated with water, can be a fiercely lonely time. The main holidays of all the major religions fall in these deepest of dark days. Family time can bring up old hurts and make us feel disempowered or fearful. Turning our fear into hope, trust, faith, or courage is the balm we need to help us thrive through this season.

From the water of winter, we're going to emerge into the solidity of spring. In water we plant a seed, a desire. We choose a reality, and with that choice, we collapse the quantum field (for each particular situation), meaning that once we make a choice, we have also chosen not to take all the other options. We make one choice and go down that one road, and hence comes the fear—fear of choosing a reality and then feeling as if we're losing "choice" because we have already made one.

Hope and faith are counterbalancers for the fear of water. Hope is the precursor to faith, which is a dogged certainty. Hope is also the first step toward water coming out of its shell. In that deep and darkest water saturation, the imbalanced fear that often leads to depression is a feeling of awfulness about life in general—this is how life is, it will always be like this, and it will never get better—or the fear that if we move and do something, anything, this whole fragile world will fall apart. What was once so perfect will end. If we even hope for a moment, we open ourselves up to the doubt or the loss. But it is also that very wholeness of hope that makes it so powerful—the fact that it contains the gains as well as the losses, the possibilities of both.

In the depth of water, if you can hope for one small thing, it can help pull you out of the water. That's what you need when you're in that deep. If you can ignite a small possibility of hope, you can shine a light into the situation, and that light will perform a sort of photosynthesis on your problem and start to transform it into material form—the wood, the next element—so you can come out of the water and into the physical. Because hope also holds the possibility of failure, when you are stuck in the depth of water, or depression, it is still possible to bring in hope. It doesn't require the full-fledged belief and resilience that faith does. It only requires you to believe that the possibility for change exists. That is the power of hope. It is a tiny ray of sunshine. And it can help you transform anything.

The emotional and psychological hallmark of the water element, along with fear, is depression, with all its other attributes: lack of desire, lack of will, lack of excitement and joy for the world, a tendency to withdraw and to be suspicious of others. Water people, when out of balance, tend to isolate, which exacerbates the feeling of being alone in the world with no support.

Too much water leads to depression; not enough water leads to lack of movement and the flow of life, lack of decision making, and lack of will and deep commitment—a disconnection from life. When out-of-balance, water people internalize, they go under water. They become detached, wishy-washy, and stagnant. They have no courage to get going, no energy to take momentum forward. If they have too much water, they don't have enough direction and end up wasting their energy. It's like a flash flood going through. This leads to kidney depletion and adrenal burnout. It's a depletion of the life force energy.

In winter we must choose our seed, our vow, our path carefully, and with intention and discernment. And then we bathe it in the water to germinate it.

The Physiology of Water

Physiologically, the water element governs the teeth, the bones, and all the fluids of the body except for blood. When you break it down into its two main organ complexes, Kidney and Bladder, you get even deeper into the power of water. Bladder, which is the longest meridian in the body, governs the nervous system. This is of tremendous importance, as Bladder goes along the spinal column twice, once along a path that corresponds to the physical body and once along a path that corresponds to the emotional body. Keeping Bladder strong is key to a healthy nervous system. Kidney is responsible for detoxing the body (along with the liver) and is also aligned with the fight-flight-freeze response in the body, with its close association to the adrenal glands. It is also a part of a healthy sexual and reproductive system in both men and women. The energy of Kidney both starts our energetic flow and also grounds us. In fact, one of the best things you can do for your health is to walk barefoot on the earth, stimulating the Kidney energy and connecting with the electrical grounding and healing energy of the earth.

When water is out of balance, we can feel a variety of symptoms. By bringing water into balance, oftentimes other challenges are also brought in line due to the powerful "start-up" force of the water element. In fact, when using techniques to balance the meridians, we always start working with Kidney (or whichever yin meridian closest to Kidney presents as imbalanced). By starting the application of energy here, it follows the Five Element Wheel with the energy, opening up and balancing all the other yin meridians. The natural body intelligence balances out each meridian, bringing more energy where there is a lack and pushing through and clearing out energy that is in excess. This is the power of water. It is the start. It is the place where all potential lies, coiled up, like the kanda energy of kundalini at the base of the spine.

In balancing water, we have to take into consideration all the parts of ourselves that are at play here. This is the most inactive time of year for flora and fauna in the Northern Hemisphere. It is a time of deep rest and repose, of turning inward. Words such as *hibernation* come to mind. It is the deepest yin of the yins. No time during our annual cycle is more interior, introspective, and connected to source as the water time. In the best case, we take this time also to turn inward, to look back on the year that is just passing and reflect on how we fared. It is the time to tune in deeply and to choose consciously the seeds we want to plant for the next season. It can be a time of deep healing and deep inner seeing, a time to get in touch with our own intuitive powers and our powers of self-determination, and a time to regroup and heal on a deep interior level from the roughness of the outer world. It is a great opportunity, if we take it, to reflect on what is working and on what needs to change in our lives. It is a time of great and simple beauty in the world, where things are reduced to their essence and the elegance of underlying structure is revealed.

Water time can also be a scary time. The earth itself is hidden, and there is a feeling of being disconnected from what sustains us. Feeling alone and frightened can regress us to feelings of childhood, when we didn't have control or power in our own lives. If we can tap into the powerful truth—instead of run from it—that we really don't have control of our lives, this understanding can finally free us to see more clearly where we can exercise our will to positive effect and where we must simply surrender.

In terms of the physical body and how you will support water in your EMYoga practice, it is the fetus and the baby. It is all fetal position and tucked in close, swaddled, squatting, and smallening the body. This practice is about beginnings—squats, gentle twists, forward bends. It is about inward looking to gain perspective and then beginning to turn out to the world again, which takes courage. There is also the pulse, or in Sanskrit the *spanda*, that is inherent in the water element. Each element has an action that helps propel it forward into the next element. For water, moving toward wood, it is this spanda, or pulsation. Thus, you will start with the small balled-up form and move outward toward opening, like the spouting of a seed. This also mimics physiologically the movement of fear toward courage.

The sounds that are made are the first breathiness of simply blowing air out of the mouth, maybe born from a cough, a sneeze, or the mother blowing kisses to the new baby's face. The sound of blowing through the lips is the sound that activates and thus heals both the Kidney and the Bladder. It is a sound almost identical to the first word ever attributed to the name of God: *huuuu* (sounds like *you*, not *who*).

Water Properties

Governs	Teeth, bones, all fluids in the body except blood
Season	Winter
Meridians	Kidney (yin), Bladder (yang)
Archetypes	The baby, the philosopher, the king
Main Emotions	Challenging: Fear Balancing: Courage, hope, faith

The EMYoga Water Practice

1 Wake Up

Stand for the Wake Up. One of the main needs of the body is the ability to expand outward and to contract inward. Most of us, as we age, can do the expansion, but the contraction becomes harder and harder. So we start the practice by "shaking out" the body, getting it to start moving energetically from this expansive perspective, and then slowly moving into the smaller and smaller. See the online video and page 78 for the Wake Up practice instructions.

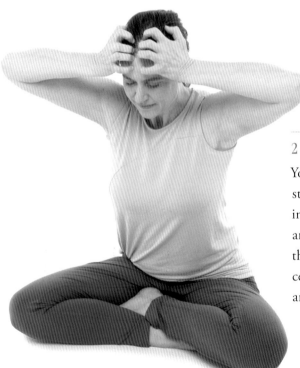

2 Crown Pull

You can do the next two moves standing or sitting. Press your fingers into the center of your forehead, and with a strong pressure pull them apart. Continue this along the center seam of your skull all the way around to your neck.

3 Spinal Flush

Continue this pressure with your fingertips down your neck and down the sides of your spine until you can't reach any farther. Then pull your hands, with pressure, up over your shoulders. Continue to massage down your sternum, between your breasts, to where the ribs meet. Drag your fingers around to your back again, and then massage your thumbs down either side of your spine to your coccyx. Brush off your back three times. See the online video.

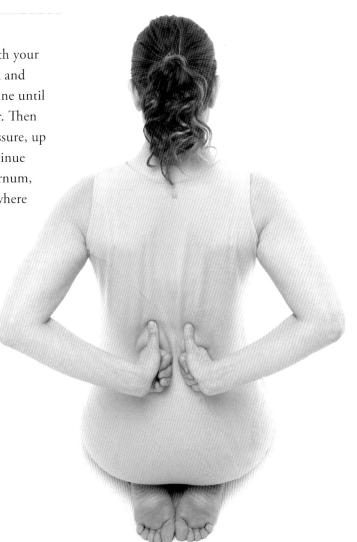

4 Calf Clear in Cobbler

Baddha Konasana

Come to sit, and place your feet loosely together, knees out to the sides. Leave space to reach the soles of your feet with your fingers. Stay in this position as you do the practices described next.

Kidney 1 (K1) Pulse

Find the slight indent where the ball of your big toe meets the ball of your second toe (K1). Press in deeply with your thumbs. Press and release this point deeply several times.

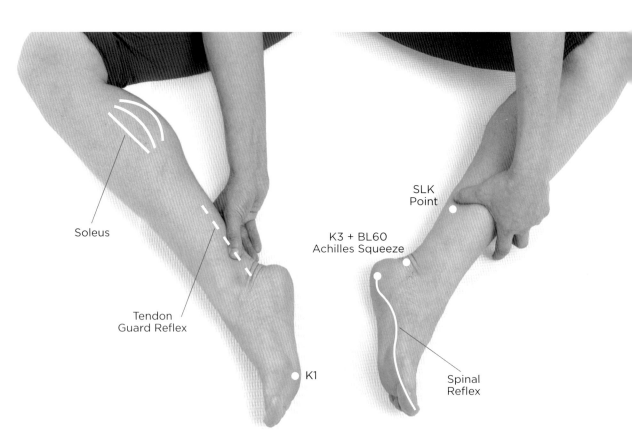

Soleus

Tendon Guard Reflex

K1

SLK Point

K3 + BL60 Achilles Squeeze

Spinal Reflex

Clear Foot Gates

Starting in the middle of both feet, massage down the tendons between your metatarsal bones (the long bones in your feet that become your toes). Massage on both sides of your feet by reaching under your toes with your fingers and pinch off in the gullies between your toes. Then massage down the bones of your toes and pinch off the tip of each toe.

Spine Reflex on Feet

Massage down the outside bones of your upward-facing feet, from the edge of your big toes, up over the side arches, to behind your ankle bones.

Achilles Squeeze

Note: Do not do this if you are pregnant.

Squeeze and/or massage both sides of your Achilles tendon.

Tendon Guard Reflex and Soleus Massage

Massage up your Achilles tendon and continue deep massage up the widest, fleshiest part of your calf.

Spleen-Liver-Kidney (SLK) Point Massage

Note: Do not do this if you are pregnant.

Find the sore point about a hand's width up from the upward-facing center of your Achilles tendon. This is a junction of Spleen, Liver, and Kidney meridians. Massage it deeply.

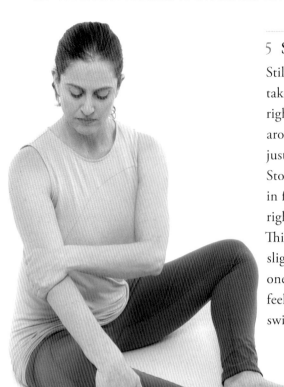

5 Sedate Triple Warmer, Seated

Still seated in baddha konasana, take a slight twist toward the right. Now wrap your right hand around your right leg, holding just below your knee (covering Stomach 36). Wrap your left hand in front of your torso around your right elbow (Triple Warmer 10). This will cause your body to twist slightly toward the right. Hold one to three minutes or until you feel the synchronized pulse. Then switch sides.

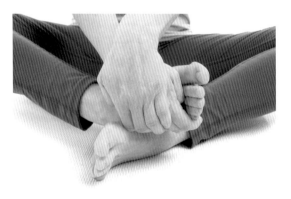

6 Control Points for Triple Warmer

Snug both feet in closer so you can reach them with your hands. You may need to put a bit of padding under your feet. Hold your right foot on the side edge of your pinky toe (Bladder 66). Hold your right hand with your left hand, covering the base of your fourth finger (Triple Warmer 2).

7   Blowing Out the Candle

See page 86 for full instructions and the online video.

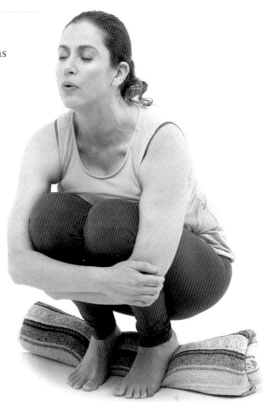

8   Cat-Cow

Come forward onto your hands and knees. Inhale and lift your spine into an arch. Exhale and sink your spine into a hammock. Do this several times. Take a few breaths to arch your spine side to side as well, making the body into a crescent moon shape.

9 All Fours to Child's Pose

Balasana

Come back to neutral on all fours. Inhale here, then exhale and lower your butt to your heels into child's pose. Inhale and come back up to all fours. Do this three times. This is a perfect pose to introduce or practice using mula bandha (see page 73). On the exhale, engage the bandha as you sit back onto your heels. Repeat this three times.

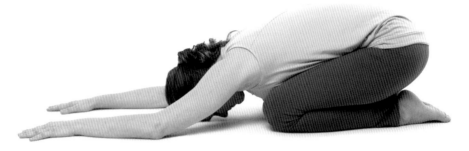

10 Child's Pose Weaving Heaven

Start in child's pose. On an inhale, lift your body up to stand on your knees with your arms up overhead. Exhale and weave your arms back and forth in front of your body as you release into child's pose. Inhale to all fours. Exhale to child's pose. Do this three times. Feel the energy and your breath moving in you like a wave. See the online video.

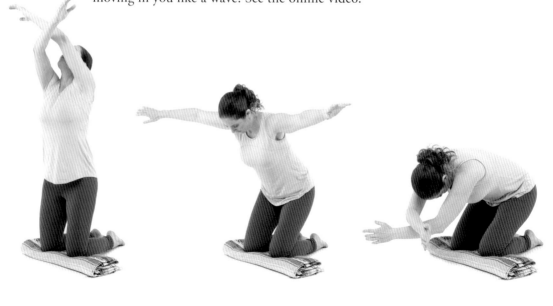

11 Bean with Head Heal

Come slightly up and forward from child's pose and walk your elbows forward. Rest your head in your hands, with the heels of your hands on your cheekbones and your palms over your eye sockets. Breathe here for as long as feels good. Now lift your head slightly and press your thumbs into the inside upper corners of your eyes, where they meet your nose. This is the first point on the Bladder meridian, the start of the longest meridian, which runs twice down your spine. Hold here and breathe for several moments. Release back into child's pose; bring your hands into fists behind you and deeply and strongly massage your kidneys, at your low back, just below your bottom ribs.

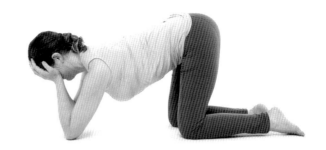

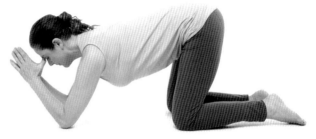

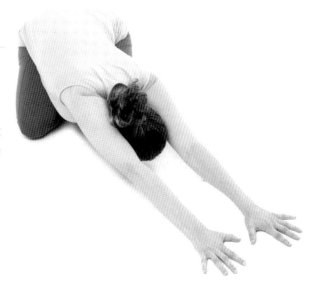

12 Child's Pose Side Stretch

From child's pose, lengthen your arms out in front of you and walk them slightly to the right, stretching your whole side body. Repeat on the other side.

13 Rabbit with Heel Pulse

Sasangasana

From child's pose, cup your hands over your heels. Press your fingers in and massage your heels and bottoms of your feet, which will release stored shock from your body. Use the pressure of your fingertips pressing into your heels to pull your body back as you lean forward with your weight coming to the crown of your head. You can hold behind your knees if that feels better. Stretch your whole spine. Release back into child's pose.

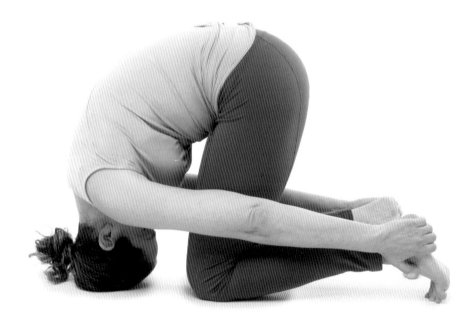

14 All Fours to Child's Pose to All Fours to Downward Dog

Adho Mukha Svanasana

From child's pose, inhale to all fours and exhale to child's pose. Inhale to all fours and exhale to downward dog. Repeat this three to five times.

15 Knees-Chest-Chin—Inchworm

Ashtanga Namaskara

From downward dog, lower your knees, then your chest, then your chin to the floor. Your butt will be up in the air. Make sure your elbows are tucked in to your side body. Try to breathe as deeply and smoothly as you can. Hold for five breaths. Then bring your weight into your hands and bring yourself forward, and release flat onto the floor.

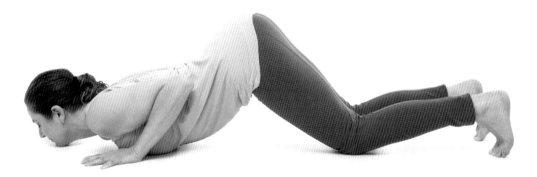

16 Triple Warmer Rock

Lower onto your belly. Make a pillow with your hands and rest your forehead on them. Rock your hips side to side. This releases the fight-or-flight response in your body by calming the Triple Warmer meridian.

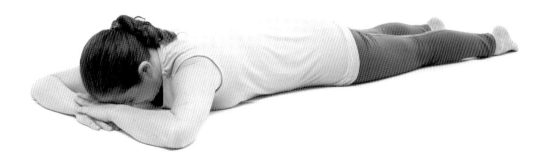

17 Cobra

Bhujangasana

Bring your hands under your shoulders and slowly start to lift your torso up using the muscles in your back to curl into a backbend before you engage your arms. Come up as high as feels comfortable. Strongly engage the muscles of your butt and legs. Legs stay on the floor. Hold three to five breaths. Release down to your belly with your head on your hands and rock your hips side to side.

18 Locust

Shalabasana

Lie on your belly. Lift your head, neck, shoulders, and arms off the floor, and then lift both legs from the floor, engaging your leg and butt muscles strongly. Arms can be straight out in front of you, out to the sides, or along your body with your palms facing out. Hold for five breaths and return to the floor, head on your hands, and rock your hips.

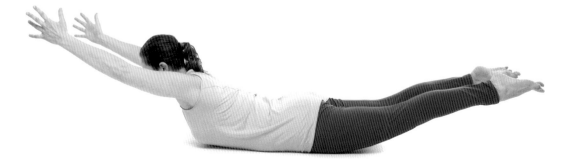

19 Foot to Butt

Still lying on your belly, come up on your elbows. Reach back and press your foot with the same-side hand down toward your butt. Make sure to press both hip bones down to the floor. Hold for several breaths, stretching the front of your quadriceps. Switch sides.

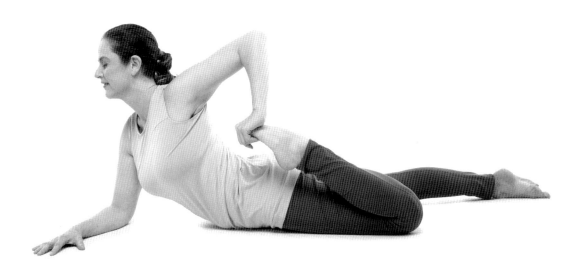

20 Cat-Cow

Come onto your hands and knees and do a few more rounds of cat-cow to release your back. Arch and concave your back in conjunction with your breath.

21 Camel with Water Hold

Ustrasana

Come to stand on your knees on some extra padding. Lift your heart center up. Bring your hands into Triple Warmer/Heart mudra (thumbs in your heart center, fingertips in the hollow at the base of your throat). Keep your hips pressing forward, as much in line with your knees as you can. Extend your right arm up and over your head to come behind you. With your thumb and your bent index finger, squeeze strongly on either side of your Achilles tendon on your right foot—thumb on the outside, index finger on the inside. *Note: Do not massage your Achilles tendon if you are pregnant. The points on the Achilles tendon are contraindicated for pregnancy.*

Now extend your left arm up and over and hold the other ankle the same way, strongly pinching your Achilles tendon between your thumb and index finger. Hold for three to five breaths.

To release, reverse the pose. Sweep your left hand over your head and back to your chest, pressing your thumb into your heart center, fingertip in throat hollow. Actively press your body up into your thumb to keep the integrity of the pose while you release your right hand, sweeping it up and over to meet your left hand in Triple Warmer/Heart mudra. Sit back on your heels with your hands in your lap and close your eyes. Repeat this pose one or two more times. You can also do one side at a time. And experiment with having your arms outwardly rotated (thumbs on the outside of Achilles) or inwardly rotated (thumbs on the inside of Achilles).

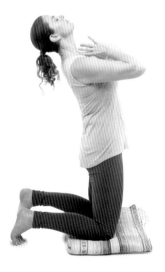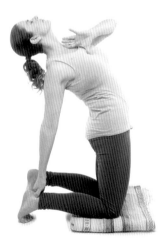

22 Three-Point Kidney: Sedate in Seated Spinal Twist

Ardha Matsyendrasana

Start in a seated position, legs stretched out in front. Bring your right knee up so your right foot is flat on the floor and cross your left leg under your right. (You can also keep your right leg on the calf side of your left leg if you can't cross it over.) Inhale and lengthen your left arm up and extend it past your right knee to reach your left foot. (You can use either hand to hold your left foot, depending on how deeply you like to go into this pose). Place whichever thumb is reaching your left foot to hold under the ball of your foot (Kidney 1) (see photo for the points for all three Kidney poses). Wrap your other fingers around your big toe, touching the base of your big toenail on the inside edge (Liver 1). Hold these points lightly for two to three minutes.

As you inhale, continue lengthening your spine upward; as you exhale, deepen the twist. Bring your focus to your hand holding your left foot.

Continue holding a few more breaths, and then release the pose; take a gentle counterstretch to the other side, then take the pose to the other side.

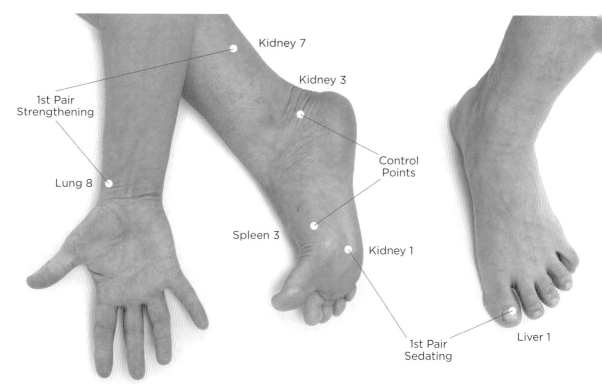

Kidney 7

Kidney 3

1st Pair
Strengthening

Control
Points

Lung 8

Spleen 3

Kidney 1

1st Pair
Sedating

Liver 1

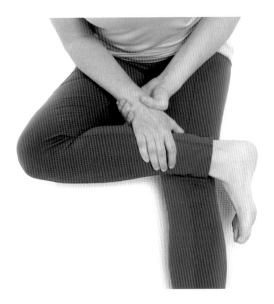

23 Strengthen Kidney: Half-Ankle to Knee

Ardha Agnistambhasana

Starting in a seated position, with your legs stretched out in front, cross your right ankle over your extended straight left leg, directly above your knee. Bring your right hand to "cuff" over your mid-calf (Kidney 7). Bring your left hand to "cuff" under your wrist (Lung 8). Lean forward from your hips and hold one to two minutes. Switch sides.

24 Control Kidney: Cobbler

Baddha Konasana

Bring the soles of your feet together, knees apart. Bring your thumbs into the centers of the upward-facing exposure of your Achilles tendons (Kidney 3); bring your fingertips to rest on the sides of the balls of your feet as shown (Spleen 3). Lean forward into the pose, bending from your hips, not your waist. Stay for one minute. *Tip:* You can do all three holds for Kidney strengthening in cobbler's pose.

25 Seated Cortisol Breath

Take a comfortable seat with a bit of padding under your butt to raise your hips off the floor slightly, and allow your spine to easily settle into its natural curves. Take a few deep, clearing, and centering breaths. Now inhale deeply, as much as you can, and pull your belly in. At the top of the inhale, when it feels as if you can't inhale any more, sniff in three more quick breaths. Exhale completely. Now inhale completely and exhale all the air out until it seems as if you have no air left in your lungs. Again, keep your belly pulled in. Exhale three quick exhales, pushing out three more puffs of air. Inhale completely. Do this again, both directions, two more times. This helps to balance the cortisol levels in your body. See the online video.

26 Cortisol Thread Thru

Bring one hand to your crown. Bring your other hand one inch below your belly button. Open your thumb and middle finger two inches so they cover the points one inch below and one inch to the side of your belly button. Inhale and pull the top arm up, then exhale, lowering that hand back to the crown and pulling your other hand out from your belly. Do this back and forth, as if you are pulling a piece of thread up and down between the crown and the cortisol points on your belly. Repeat several times. This balances cortisol levels. See the online video.

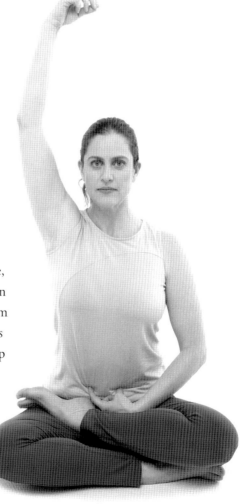

27 Moving Bridge with Water Neurolymphatic Clear

Dwi Pada Pitham

See full instructions on page 94 and in the online video of the Essential EMYoga practice.

While resting from moving bridge, use a very strong pressure to massage the neurolymphatic points for Kidney, Bladder, and other points, as shown. Shake your hands off. Exhale through your mouth, making the sound *whooo*. If it feels good to you, come up again into bridge for five more breaths.

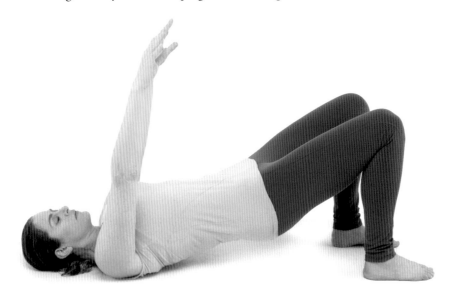

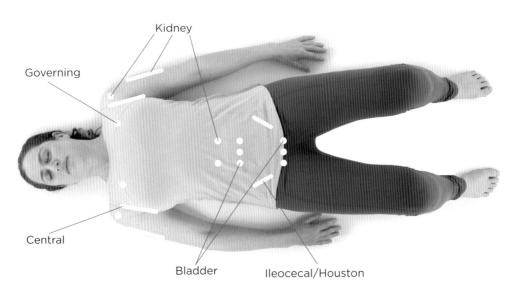

28 Supported Shoulder Stand or Legs Up the Wall with Electrics

Sarvangasana or Viparita Karani
See full directions on page 96 and in the online video.

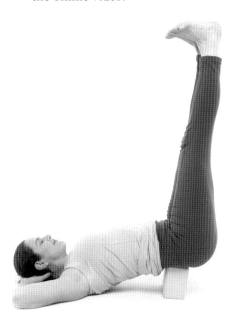

29 Laughing Baby with Calf Massage, Then Kidney 1 Pulse

Ananda Balasana

Lie on your back, fold your knees into your chest, release your low back, and breathe deeply. Start to lift your feet into the sky for laughing baby, and as you do so, massage again your soleus muscle (the fleshiest part of the calf), where it starts to thin out (the tendon guard reflex), and your Achilles tendon. *Note: Do not massage your Achilles tendon if you're pregnant.* End with your knees bent toward your armpits and your feet facing the sky. Hold on to your feet and press your fingers into Kidney 1. Pulse this point a few times, then hold, pressing into Kidney 1 with your hands as your knees descend deeper toward your armpits. Stay here for several breaths.

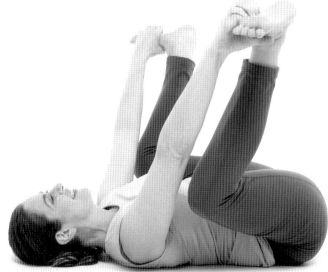

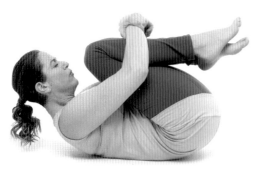

30   Blowing Out the Candle, Reclining

Lie on your back and hug your knees into your chest. Inhale and lift your head up to your knees. Exhale with an audible *whoooo*, and release your head back down to the floor. Do this three times.

31   Body Cross

Lie on your back with knees bent, feet on the floor. Make a large X on your body. First, squeeze the muscle on the top of one shoulder, then "slice" through your body to the opposite hip. Make an X by repeating the same squeeze and slice on the other side. Do each side again.

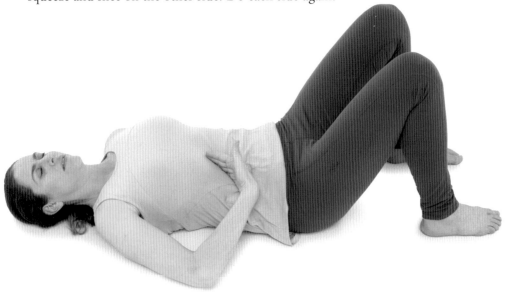

32 Hook Up

Place one finger in your belly
button, one finger at your third eye,
and press both in and pull up. Take
three full deep breaths, in your nose
and out your mouth.

33 Savasana Prep with Water Neurovascular Reflex Points Hold

Lie on your back with your legs slightly apart. You can put a rolled blanket
under your knees and a block under your top arm for support if you like.
Before you fully surrender to the pose, bring one hand to cover your forehead,
as if you were taking your temperature. Bring your other hand over the lower
curve of your skull. Hold here for at least a minute or as long as feels good to
you. This helps release the emotional residue of water: fear. You can bring to
mind something you're working with, or just allow the hold to do its magic.
When you feel ready, release your arms down to your sides.

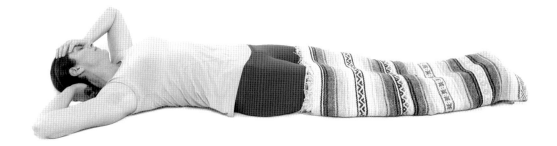

34   Savasana

Let the body relax completely. Let your trace of awareness rest on any new sensations or feelings that are occurring in your body. Don't try to identify them; just let your awareness rest with these newly awakened energies. They may appear as color, light, warmth, heat, sound, or even smell or taste. Remain here for five to fifteen minutes.

35   Pranayama: Sama Vritti

Come to a comfortable, supported seat. *Sama vritti* means "equal breath." The goal is to make the length of the inhale equal to the length of the exhale. This practice helps bring disciplined awareness to the breath; it also conditions your lungs and starts to build their capacity.

To help you equalize your inhale and exhale, put a count to your breath. Slowly and evenly, count one, two, three, four as you inhale, and then exhale to the same number of counts until the inhale and exhale are even. As your breath capacity deepens, the count will naturally get longer; just continue to make both the inhale and exhale the same length. This breath helps bring your body and nervous system into balance and brings more equanimity to your practice. You can do this pranayama at the start or end of your practice.

36   Meditation

Sit and listen for five to twenty minutes. First listen to the farthest sounds, and then listen to sounds closer and closer in to your body. Then listen to the sounds coming from inside your own body. Finally, listen or feel your own heartbeat. Keep your awareness here for the remainder of your meditation.

6

Wood

Spring. The season of rebirth. The buds start to appear on the trees, flowers push up from the earth, sometimes when it's still covered in snow. New beginnings, warmth, and more light remind us of our resilience, of the constant cycles, that the dawn always comes after the dark.

The element of spring is wood. Life returns and in a seeming instant the gray and brown world is lit with a million colorful buds. Spring holds much within its season.

The two meridians in wood are Liver and Gallbladder. It's fitting in that the liver is the only organ in the body that can rebuild itself even if 80 percent of the tissue is destroyed. This is the very definition of renewal. The liver is responsible for removing toxins, creating hormones, and cleaning the blood. Energetically it is responsible for the smooth flow of chi, or life-force energy in the body. It's also in charge of the smooth flow of blood through the body, and as a result of those two dynamics, the smooth flow of emotions. If your emotions aren't able to move through you, they become stuck and cause myriad problems. So it is important that the wood element is balanced, giving you the strength to deal with whatever comes at you.

The gallbladder is responsible for helping the body digest fats, the most important nutrient in the body. Every single cell is cased in fat. Your brain is more than 60 percent fat. Your body is encased in a layer of protective fat. Fat helps you create healthy hormones. And fat is necessary for those hormones to be utilized (more on fat in part 3). Fats are necessary and also challenging for the body to digest, and they rely on the enzymes that the gallbladder releases to do so. Although the gallbladder is a small organ, it has an important and difficult job.

The Psychology of Wood

Aside from what the liver and gallbladder do physiologically, they are incredibly important to the psychology of the body. The main emotion correlated to wood is anger. This is the anger of the teenager who doesn't yet know their place in the world, who feels powerless. It is also sometimes considered to be the anger of the toddler, not understanding why things can't always be the way they want them to be, propelling them into a tantrum. This anger doesn't only come when we are children or teenagers, although those are clearly times of unfocused anger, but the anger comes whenever we feel that same powerlessness—that same uncertainty about who we are and what our place is in the world. It is the anger over all the unfairness in the world that we feel we can't affect.

To balance that, we need to bring out our assertiveness and courage. Although courage is a water balancer, it is also in play here, in the neighboring element. We need to have the courage of our convictions and then the assertiveness to stand our ground. We must also come into contact with our innate feelings of worth—that we have a right to our opinions, that we have certain inalienable rights, and that we accept those rights along with the responsibilities they confer. It isn't acceptable to break a law in order to right a wrong. This is an important distinction because the power of anger can lead to righteousness if it isn't channeled correctly. Conversely, many of us feel unworthy of going out and getting what we want. Perhaps you were told as a child that you would never amount to anything and you've internalized that, so you find now, as an adult, you're constantly making excuses for yourself. Marianne Williamson sums this up perfectly in her book *A Return to Love*: "Our deepest fear is not that we are inadequate. Our deepest fear is that we are powerful beyond measure. It is our light, not our darkness that most frightens us. We ask ourselves, 'Who am I to be brilliant, gorgeous, talented, fabulous?' Actually, who are you not to be? You are a child of God. Your playing small does not serve the world."[1]

We can stop ourselves from action if we don't feel we have a right to take our place in the world. The truth is this: every tree has its place in the forest.

There is no need to make excuses for yourself. Your goal is to discover your inner strengths and gifts and then to share them with the world, increasing the light. As Martha Graham said: "There is a vitality, a life force, an energy, a quickening that is translated through you into action, and because there is only one of you in all time, this expression is unique. And if you block it, it will never exist through any other medium and will be lost."[2]

Taking your place at the table and in the world isn't a matter of greed but rather revealing the lie we've been fed about limited resources. It is not resources that are in short supply, but imagination, love, compassion, and caring. Perhaps you are the one who will fill a void in the matrix of transformation from a culture of consumption and disposability to one of conservation and collectivity. But if you don't step up to the plate, that job goes unfilled and undone. Perhaps it is a matter of turning your rage and anger that the world is unfair into the assertion that you have an answer and will make yourself heard. This is the benefit of transmuting anger. It can be a powerful motivator if you can take the fuel behind it and transform it into constructive action. Rosa Parks could have gotten angry, yelled, or stomped around. Instead, she simply and strongly asserted her right to sit on the bus and in doing so sparked a revolution.

In wood, we take the seeds that we chose in water and prune the sprouts. They are starting to burst forth. They are starting to take shape into their final form, and it is during this time that we can tweak them. Like thinning the garden bed to make room for things to grow really big, wood is the season in which we pull out the choices that we don't like and add more fertilizer to the ones we do.

This is the time we start to assert ourselves. We know ourselves deeper. We know what we like, what we stand for, and what we are willing to die for.

The Physiology of Wood

The wood practice is focused on standing poses. Learning how to stand our ground requires strengthening the physical muscles to do so. It also requires a release of the anger that destabilizes us. I think of the quote on my friend's refrigerator: "Anger is like drinking poison and hoping the other person dies." We can think of our anger as compostable instead. We put in all the scraps, the junk, the unwanted, the rage, the pain, the hatred. Let the heat of those emotions out, and the anger cooks down into nutrients for the growing plants. It is a transformation of the "junk" to the gold. In a similar way, we need to get the "junk" out of our emotional system so that we create space for the growing plants—our own desires and our gifts to the world.

We also have to maintain flexibility as we grow. Without flexibility, the first storm to come through will rip out our tree at the root or break the trunk in half. We have to learn how to flex with the storms. This requires strength, stability, and movement of the spine. As we strengthen wood and prepare to move toward the coming season of fire, the movement is a gentle waving of the spine, like a weeping willow or the strength and flexibility of bamboo. This also gives us more access to the energetics of the core, which need to be strong enough to support us on our paths.

The sound that directly taps into the healing power of wood is *shhhhh*. We use that sound in Expelling the Venom (see page 87), which is the technique to get out the junk that keeps us stuck, clearing space for our true strength to emerge.

Wood Properties

Governs	Muscles, tendons, ligaments, nails
Season	Spring
Meridians	Liver (yin), Gallbladder (yang)
Archetypes	The warrior, the pioneer, the commander
Main Emotions	Challenging: Anger
	Balancing: Assertiveness

The EMYoga Wood Practice

1 Wake Up

Do the Wake Up standing, and really move in a big way to open up your body for this intense energy to easily flow through. See the online video and page 78 for instructions.

2 Liver Meridian Clear

Sit in a loose baddha konasana with the soles of your feet together, knees apart. Deeply massage up the pathway of the Liver meridian as shown. The points around your knee will generally be quite sore. Make sure to spend a bit of extra time on the sore points.

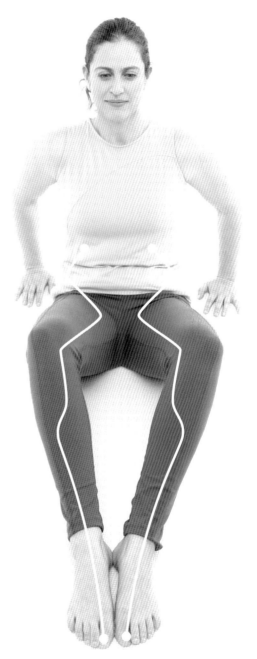

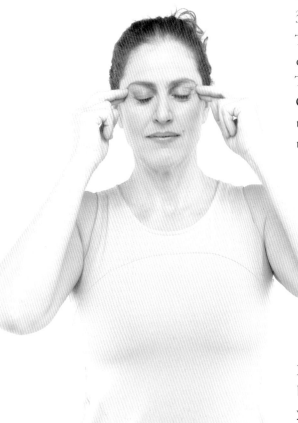

3 Gallbladder Aid

Tap strongly on the outside corners of your eyes on the orbital bone. This is the starting point of the Gallbladder meridian. Then tap on the outside edges of your fourth toe (edge toward your pinky toe as shown). This is the end point of the Gallbladder meridian. Tapping these points helps get energy moving along the meridian pathway. Now scrub your whole head, massaging deeply like you're shampooing your hair. End by smoothing several times behind your ears, as if you're pushing your hair back behind your ears. There are many Gallbladder points on the head, and this helps to open them up.

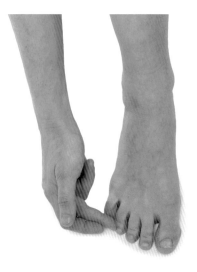

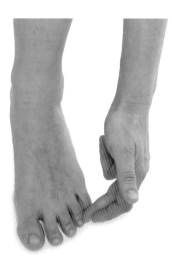

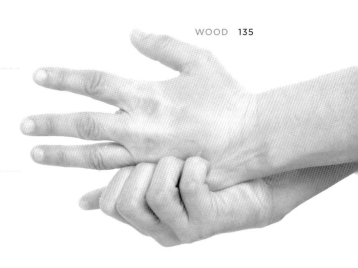

4 Clear the Gates of the Hands and Feet

See instructions on page 80.

5 Hug Knees

Roll onto your back and hug your knees into your chest. Hug your head up to your knees and take several breaths.

6 Squat

Roll forward into a squat. Put a blanket under your heels if they don't reach the floor. Stay here for several breaths.

7 Hang with Eye Socket Massage Upside-Down

Uttanasana

Allow your hips to lift up and your head, neck, and shoulders to hang down to the ground. Keep a slight bend behind your knees. Breathe here as the tension in your legs lessens and your muscles take over. Use your thumbs and fingers to strongly and carefully massage the orbital bone surrounding your eyes. Don't just quickly massage around; take your time and really feel the minute dips and hollows in the bone, massaging all the points.

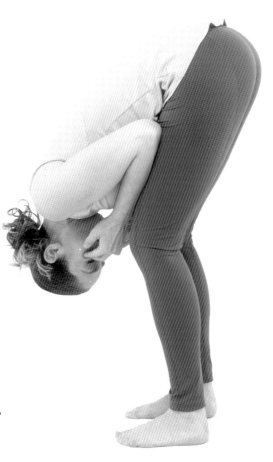

8 Bladder 1 Lift to Chair Pose

Utkatasana

From a forward bend, press your thumbs into the inside edges of your eyes close to the bridge of your nose. Gently pull your head forward and up using your thumbs, and use your arms to lift your body into chair pose. Breathe here for a moment, then continue lifting your head with your thumbs to full standing. Release your hands and cross one hand over the other on top of your heart. See the online video.

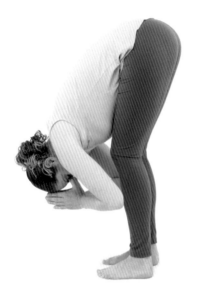
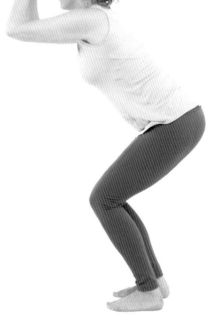

9 Mountain Pose

Tadasana

Stand tall with your hips directly over your ankles, your shoulders over your hips, and your ears over your shoulders. Roll your shoulders up, back, and down, and let your hands rest, pinky sides in, against your thighs. Remain still, quiet, and alert.

10 Arms Overhead and Side Pull

From tadasana, sweep your arms
overhead and catch your left wrist
with your right hand. Pull your
body up and over to the right. Stay
strongly anchored through your left
leg. Stay for three to five breaths.
Switch sides.

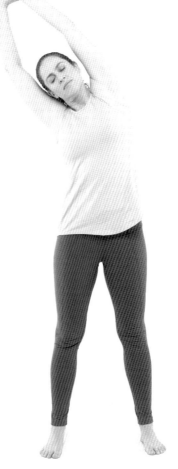

11 Yin-Yang Meridian Clear

See page 82 for full
instructions and the
online video.

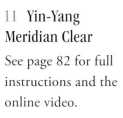

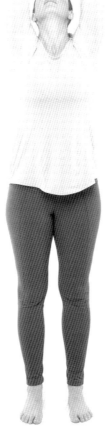

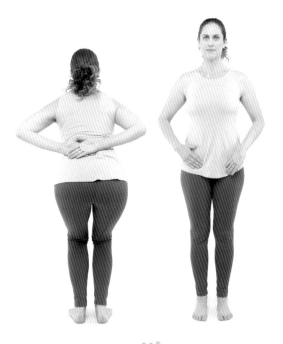

12   Chair with Penetrating Flow

Utkatasana

See complete instructions on
page 85 and the online video.

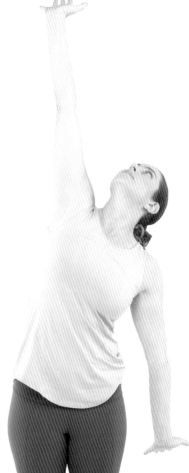

13   Connecting Heaven and Earth

From a standing position, inhale, lift
one hand up to the sky, look up, and
release one hand toward the earth,
with both palms flattened. Exhale
and bring your hands together in
front of your heart in Triple Warmer/
Heart mudra (thumbs in your heart
center, fingertips in the hollow at
the base of your throat). Inhale and
do this to the other side. Repeat two
more times each side. Make this feel
like little sprouts, or little flowers,
waking up in the morning and
stretching after a long winter's nap.
Finally, release your body into a full
forward bend. See the online video.

14 Expelling the Venom

See page 87 for full instructions
and the online video.

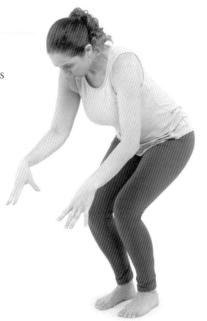

15 Tree with Triple Warmer/ Spleen Hug

Vriksasana

Come into tree pose on your right
leg. Press the left foot somewhere
along your inner leg. Make sure
your left foot is pressing against
your inner right leg, but not against
your knee. Wrap your right arm
around your waist in front of you,
and your left arm over that to
cover your opposite elbow (Triple
Warmer/Spleen hug). Activate your
standing leg strongly. Hold three
to five breaths. Release, and switch
sides or continue with the next two
poses in a mini-sequence.

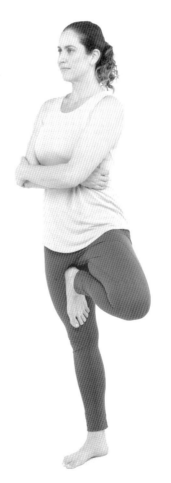

16 Warrior 1 with Triple Warmer/Spleen Hug

Virabhadrasana 1

From standing (or tree), step your left foot back and turn your foot out about thirty degrees. Bend your front knee, coming into warrior 1. Wrap your right arm around your left rib cage and actively pull your rib cage forward, then wrap your left arm over your right, cupping your elbow. Keep your shoulders down but lift your heart. Anchor your back foot and keep weight on its outside edge. Engage your leg muscles, as if you're pulling tights up. Hold three to five breaths. Repeat on the other side or continue with the next pose.

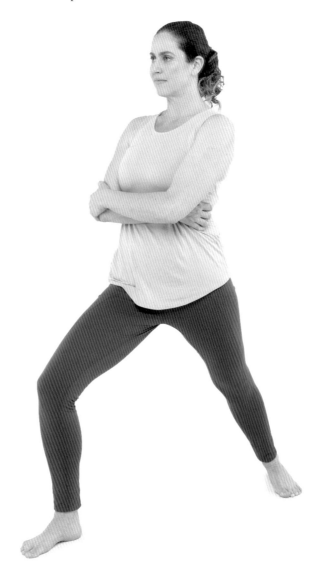

17 Warrior 3 with Triple Warmer/Spleen Hug

Virabhadrasana 3

Look forward and lift your back (left) leg up, coming into warrior 3.
Bring your back leg parallel to the floor with your toes pointing down. Hold
three to five breaths and step back to tadasana. Repeat on the other side.

Note: You can do the previous three asanas all together in a flow:
moving from tree to warrior 1 to warrior 3, all with the same arm hold
(Triple Warmer/Spleen hug); and then a second time, with arms up
overhead and then forward for the warrior poses or out to the sides,
Superman style, for warrior 3. See the online video.

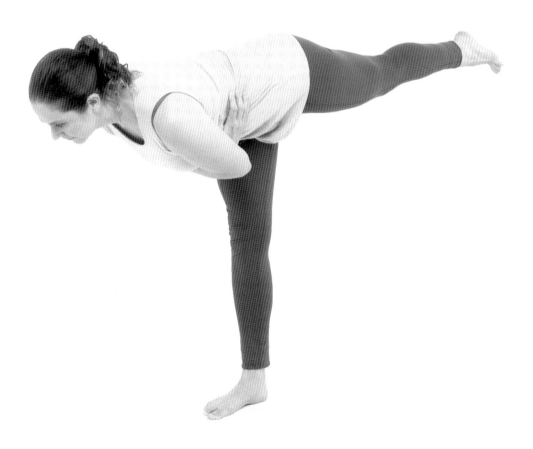

18 Schoolyard Hook Up

From standing, cross one foot over the other. Straighten your arms out in front of you, palms facing away from each other, thumbs down. Cross one hand over the other and, interlacing your fingers, bring your palms together. Scoop your hands under and up, and hug them into your body. Take three to five breaths and switch sides.

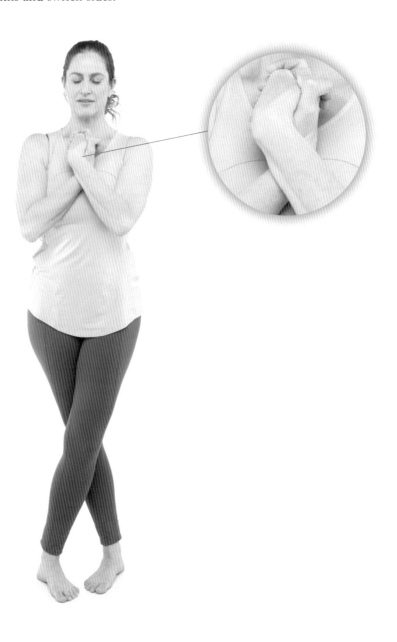

19 EMYoga Eagle

Garudasana

Come into full eagle with your left leg bent and your right leg crossed once around your left leg, or possibly twice, with your right foot hooked behind your left ankle. Sink down into your standing leg. Cross your left arm over your right arm once and possibly twice. The palms of your hands will be touching, though not exactly aligned. Lift the arms up while keeping your shoulders down. Hold three to five breaths and release by flying your arms and your legs open. Then bring your thumbs into the center of your forehead and smooth out to your temples. With your thumbs at your temples, curl your fingertips into the center of your forehead, press in, and smooth apart. Repeat the whole pose on the second side. See the online video.

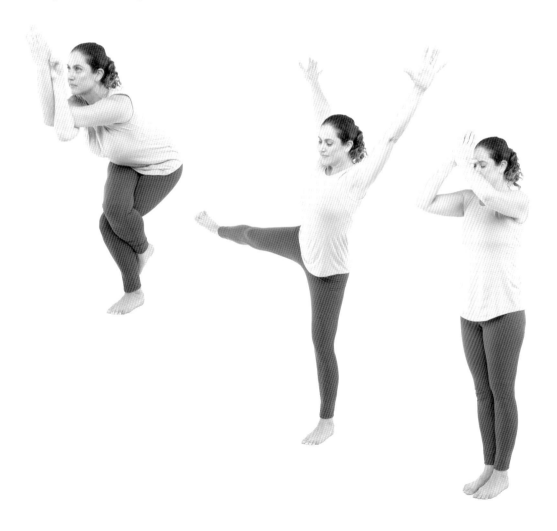

20   Expelling the Venom

Do another round of Expelling the Venom. See page 87 for full instructions and the online video.

21   Slow Squat with Squat Lunge

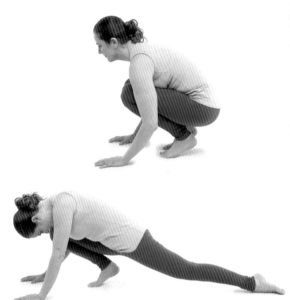

Slowly lower down into a squat. For this squat, you don't need an anchor under your heels. Stay here for several breaths. Then slowly move your left leg back into a lunge while staying as low to the ground in your squat as possible. Bring that leg back into the squat and release your right leg back into a squat lunge. Move forward and back several times, staying as low to the ground as possible, opening up your hips and groins.

22   Full Squat with Arm Extension

Malasana

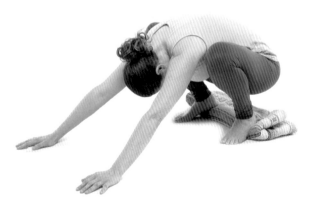

Come back into a full squat. Use padding underneath your heels to anchor yourself. In this deep squat, lean your torso forward between your legs, arms reaching out along the floor. You can use blocks or bolsters to support your arms wherever feels right. Stay here for several long slow breaths. You can shake out your legs before moving to the next pose if you need.

23 Bean with Head Heal

Release down onto your knees and walk your elbows forward. Rest your head in your hands, with the heels of your hands on your cheekbones and your palms over your eye sockets. Breathe here for as long as feels good.

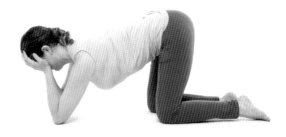

24 Slow Sit-Ups with Hook Up

See page 92 for full instructions and the online video.

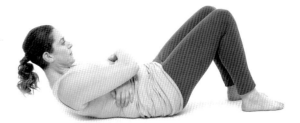

25 Moving Bridge with Wood Neurolymphatic Clear

Dwi Pada Pitham

Lie on your back with your knees bent, feet on the floor. Raise your hips and lift your arms overhead on inhale. Exhale, hips down, arms down. Repeat three to five times. Then hold up in the lifted pose three to five breaths. Release down and let your knees gently rest against each other. Deeply massage the wood neurolymphatic points shown. Exhale with an audible *shhhhh*.

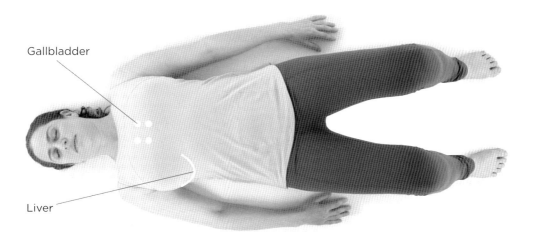

Gallbladder

Liver

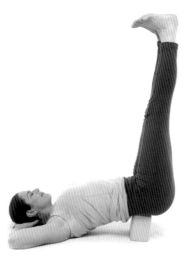

26 Supported Shoulder Stand or Legs up the Wall with Electrics

Sarvangasana or Viparita Karani

See the instructions on page 96.

27 Upward Triple Diamond: Releasing Anger and Greed

Bring the soles of your feet together, knees out to the sides. You can use padding under your knees so you can release completely. Bring your arms behind your head with your thumbs resting in the main electric points. Allow your head to rest in your hands and, if you can, let your index fingers touch. Hold here for one to two minutes, deeply breathing. If there's something you feel angry about, you can bring it to mind, or you can simply let the shape of the pose do its work, releasing anger and greed.

When you're ready to come out of the pose, press your thumbs strongly into the electric points, and then smooth them out along your neck. Finally, bring your hands to your thighs and press your thighs up with your hands instead of using your inner groin muscles.

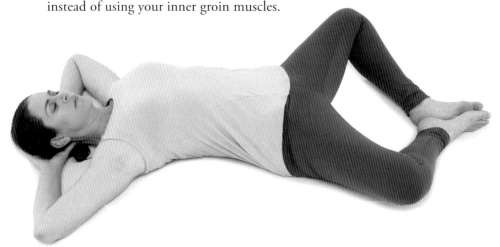

28 Hug Knees

Hug your knees into your chest and hug your head up to your knees. Hold for several breaths.

29 Lying Side Twist with Gallbladder Points Hold

See full instructions on page 98.

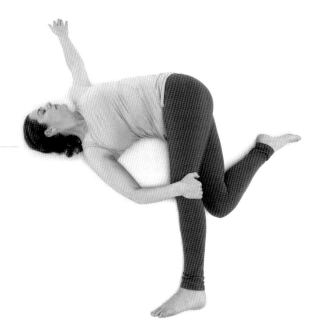

30 Savasana Prep with Wood Neurovascular Reflex Points Hold

Lie on your back in preparation for savasana. Deeply massage the third eye point, between the eyebrows. Massage your inner upper eyes and around to the outer corners. Then continue to massage your whole eye socket, using deep and controlled pressure. Lastly, rest the heels of your hands over your temples with your fingers over your forehead. This covers the wood neurovascular points and helps release any excess wood energy of anger. Breathe here until you feel relaxed, then release your arms to your sides in full savasana.

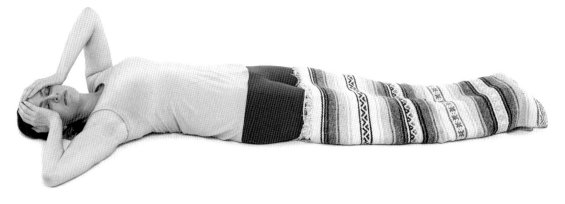

31 Savasana

Stay in savasana five to fifteen minutes, relaxing and surrendering completely.

32 Pranayama: Alternate Nostril Breath

Sit in a comfortable, supported seated position, with padding under your buttocks to allow your spine to lengthen. Bring your right hand into vishnu mudra—your first two fingers folded into your palm. Bring your thumb and fourth finger to either side of your nose. Inhale through both nostrils. Press your right thumb against the bone at the top of your right nostril, closing off your nostril completely, and exhale through your left nostril. Inhale through your left nostril, then close your left nostril with your ring finger, pressing against the bone (this is a marma point, called phana, and is a potent energy activator). Release your thumb and exhale through your right nostril. Continue this pattern: exhale, inhale, switch. Exhale, inhale, switch. Continue breathing like this for one to two minutes. Then take your last exhale through your left nostril and let your hand come back to your lap. Let your breathing adjust.

33 Meditation

Take a few deep breaths and allow yourself to settle. Bring your awareness into your spine. Start by moving your body slightly back and forth, feeling your spine in your body. Let your spine be like a tree moving gently in the breeze. Let the movements bring your awareness into your spine itself, and start to slow down the movements until you can "be" in your spine but with your body still. Visualize your brain and spinal column full of bright light. You can add a color to this if you like. See this whole area of the body illuminated. Stay here for five to twenty minutes, bathing your spine in this light. When you feel complete, do another hook up: with a finger in your belly button and at your third eye, push in and pull slightly up, three breaths, in your nose, out your mouth.

7

Fire

Have you ever had to put out a wildfire? Have you ever had to put out a house fire or a grass fire? Most people say no to this. Most people haven't been in the presence of a raging fire that requires massive resources to douse. Conversely, how many times have you struggled trying to get your woodstove lit? Or your campfire? How often have you stuffed in bundles of newspaper, trying in vain to get the soggy logs to catch?

That is the conundrum of fire. Most of us struggle in our lives for more inspiration and more joy. The anxiety we feel is often that we're not inspired about our work, our lives, our futures. We feel the opposite: overwhelmed, out of control with the amount we have to do, debilitated by the hundreds of commitments and demands placed on our time, or worse, simply bored by the repetitive tasks of life. By balancing the fire in your life, you decrease your anxiety and increase your joy and sense of inspired purpose.

Fire is the realm of the heart and of the small intestine. The heart has its own nervous system and makes decisions before fulfilling the directives of the brain. The heart has its own intelligence, and the electric field generated by the heart is the biggest of the body, extending out as much as fifteen feet from the physical body and affecting the brain patterns of people in the vicinity. The small intestine also has a strong decision-making capacity. It's constantly deciding what nutrients are good for us and needed and what to discard. The fire element is the one that makes the call on a million situations, day after day. This element is also home to the trickiest energy system in the body, Triple Warmer.

TRIPLE WARMER

Triple Warmer is a complex and dynamic energy system. In addition to feeding the adrenals and thyroid, it governs the three cavities of the torso called the "Three Burners." The low burner is at the reproductive organs; the middle burner is at the digestive organs; and the upper burner is at the heart and lungs. Triple Warmer is responsible for distributing energies among the Three Burners and helping them function in a weblike harmony. It transmits heat and moisture throughout the body. It also governs many immune activities within the body along with the fight-flight-freeze response.

The reason Triple Warmer is so important when we talk about healing is that it is often complicit in the very patterns we are trying to transform. Triple Warmer did not evolve to deal with the modern crises and constant stresses we are under, and its responses are often extreme in relation to the situation.

Because Triple Warmer is in charge of the fight-flight-freeze response, it holds an enormous amount of power over our bodies. The problem is that many events trigger a full-blown emergency response, including the inundation of chemicals and EMFs disrupting the delicate balance of our cells. This causes Triple Warmer to flood our body unnecessarily with very powerful hormones. If these hormones aren't used by the body for fighting or fleeing, they cause a continual breakdown in the body's ability to return to a neutral relaxation response, the state required for the body to heal and thrive.

When Triple Warmer loses its ability to determine what is "other" from the body, it starts to attack itself, which is the root cause of allergies and autoimmune diseases, including cancer, which is increasingly being understood as an autoimmune illness.

Triple Warmer needs to be nurtured and soothed so you don't suffer from a hair-trigger response to your environment. For this reason, many of the practices in EMYoga include techniques to calm Triple Warmer. When Triple Warmer is calm and balanced, it can then start to move into its Radiant Circuit qualities, accessing and supporting energies of healing, joy, love, and bliss. Then it gives us the feeling of calm competence that we get from nothing else. It allows us

to feel the support of the universe for our particular path and can help us reach the exalted feelings of this most precious life. Triple Warmer is a very powerful energy to have as an ally.

FOR INSTANT STRESS RELIEF, CALM TRIPLE WARMER

To quickly calm Triple Warmer (TW), lightly rest one, two, or three fingers in the hollow at the base of your throat. You can also smooth behind your ears, from the temples to the neck, 'against the flow' of TW. You'll naturally be drawn to the technique that works best for you.

Another way to calm and reprogram TW is the two point belly button hold. The belly button is the point of anchoring in to the mother, to the perfect, eternal oneness. Severing that at birth is considered our original wound, and massaging the belly button often feels soothing. Additionally, one inch below the belly button is the alarm point for TW, which alerts us when TW is overcharged. Holding these two points together anchors you in yourself, allowing the body to re-center around a new core reality of safety and peace. If you hold the belly button and the TW alarm point for 3-5 minutes, you'll feel a buzzing and 'electric' connection between them. This long hold sends the signal to TW that the original wound is okay. A womb-y sense of oneness and peace overtakes you. You'll often feel a release in your legs—a shift from the stress of 'holding it all together'—to a sense that your whole body is internally strong, held up with its own natural tensegrity, and not your muscling. This feeling is one of standing in your own power. Solid, and light as a cricket.

The Psychology of Fire

Fire is the element that makes us feel the most exalted in our lives. It is, after all, the element where love, inspiration, and joy live.

Fire people are exciting to be around. They're the ones living fully in the moment, spontaneous and ready for anything at any time, half the time instigating crazy capers. They're always bringing the sparklers to the cookout. They're the ones proposing the full-moon skinny dip. It is exhilarating to be around fires, but it can also be exhausting, and fires can exhaust themselves, leading to burnout. The challenge is to maintain that sense of excitement and wonder, but to have a slow burn so the fire doesn't burn out.

Fire is the time of life when you are building your career, putting your gifts out into the world, and becoming an adult. This means burning away or releasing the parts of you that are adolescent or immature and no longer serve the power you are meant to be in the world.

The Physiology of Fire

Fire poses are extensions and inversions, as well as heart openers and core work. The peak pose in this series is called Bringing Down the Flame, an exercise where we reeducate the fire to keep it from burning wildly around us. We guide the out-of-control energies into the wisdom of the chakras in the main channel of the spine and ultimately seat it in the belly, where it can burn bright and fuel us without destruction.

In Ayurveda, digestive fire is supremely important, as Ayurveda traces all disease back to digestion. This fire, or *agni*, in Sanskrit, is the key to overall health, when it is balanced and contained in the belly. A fire in a fire pit, or a candle, offers heat, light, and warmth; a wildfire ripping through a forest is destructive. The key for fires is to bring the raging wildfires into a controlled burning.

In fire, the goal is to increase strength so that we can navigate the challenges in our lives. The "fire in the belly" is key in this context, having fire burning brightly in our digestion system as well as our third chakra, our place of personal power. It is nearly impossible to get anything done, or manifest anything positive and lasting in this world, if we don't have a powerful and balanced third chakra. From there, we bring that strength up to the heart. If we aren't strong and balanced in the first three chakras, opening the heart can be dangerous and scary. We use fire to bridge those two, first by building and containing its power in the navel center, then letting its heat and strength rise up to the heart center to work on opening the heart to love. This strength and heart opening will find their full expression in metal, which is on the control cycle with fire. The strength and love we build here helps us withstand the challenges and difficulties in life, including loss (which is the metal element).

Heart openers are the main asanas of both fire and metal. To love and to lose and to maintain your equanimity and resilience requires an open heart.

The sound to balance the fire element is *haaaaa*. The movement to help move fire to the next element of earth is the crossover pattern. The X of the crossover pattern is the spark that propels you forward, that encourages the burning up of the excess wood you brought from the past season. Think of the primitive technique of starting a fire by rubbing two sticks together. You cross the sticks together and rub, creating friction and then a spark. With fire, you burn away all the detritus so you are left with the essence, or the core, of who you are. Balancing the four meridians in fire brings the heart and mind into balance.

Note: Within the fire practice is the protocol for sedating Triple Warmer (number 28 in the sequence below). However, this can be used outside of the practice any time you need a first-aid intervention for virtually anything. If you stub your toe, feel anxious, or get a shock, sedate Triple Warmer. If someone is upset or hurt and you don't know what to do, sedate Triple Warmer on them. The only time *not* to sedate Triple Warmer is if someone is going into anaphylactic shock from a bee sting or some other trigger. Then you want Triple Warmer to be at its full force!

Fire Properties

Governs	Blood vessels
Season	Summer
Meridians	Heart (yin), Small Intestine (yang), Circulation-Sex (yin), Triple Warmer (yang)
Archetypes	The wizard, the lover
Main Emotions	Challenging: Anxiety, panic, overwhelm Balancing: Inspiration, joy

The EMYoga Fire Practice

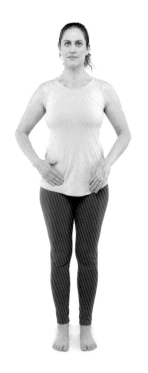

1 Wake Up

Start with a standing Wake Up. See the online video and page 78 for complete instructions.

2 Penetrating Flow

Stand in tadasana. Rub your hands in circles on your low back, then flatten them and smooth them around to your groin. Flip your hands back and forth over the edge of your pubic bone where it meets the upper thigh, then continue to smooth your hands up over your body, over your chest, and cup your hands around your mouth, making three audible exhales.

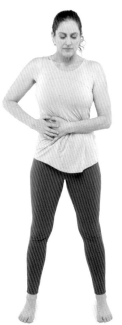

3 Belt Flow

Bring both hands to your right waist as far as possible, even slightly around to your back. Press in firmly, and smooth both hands around to your left waist. Release the hands and go back to your far-right waist. Again, press deeply and firmly across your belly to your left waist. Do this one more time. At the last arrival to your left waist, smooth your hands down the outside of your left leg and off your pinky toe. Hang over for a moment, then come up, tracing Spleen (see page 81). Repeat on the other side. See the online video.

4 Standing Straddle Twist

Parsva Prasarita Padottanasana

Step into a wide stance—with your
feet about three feet apart—feet
parallel. Inhale and bring your arms
out to your sides. Exhale and sweep
your right hand down to your left
foot. Inhale and come back up to
standing. Exhale and sweep your
left hand down to your right foot.
Inhale and come back up to standing.
Repeat three times, each side. After
the third time on the second side, stay
hanging over in the center of your
legs. Breathe here and slowly walk
your feet back to downward dog.
Take a few breaths here before
moving into the next pose.

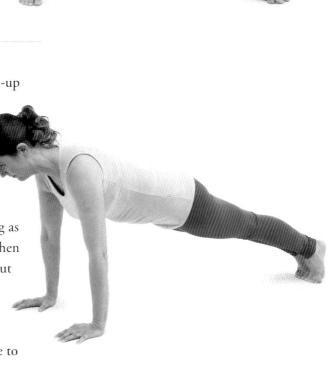

5 Long Hold Plank

Come into plank, a high push-up
position. Make sure your
hands are directly under
your shoulders. You can
let your knees come to
the floor if you cannot
stay in plank. Hold five to
ten breaths, eventually holding as
long as one to two minutes. Then
lower down to the floor and put
one hand over the other with
your top hand *palm up*. Rest
your forehead in your palm
and rock your hips side to side to
release Triple Warmer.

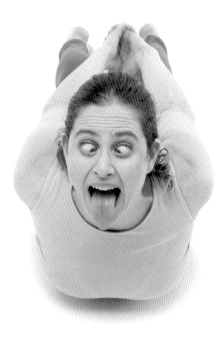

6 Low Cobra with Lion Face

Bhujangasana

From lying on your belly, lift your arms, head, neck, and shoulders. Legs stay on the floor. Engage your leg, back, and stomach muscles. Hold three to five breaths. Release, bring your hands to stack in front of you and rest your head on your hands. Rock your hips side to side. Repeat two times. On the last time, stick out your tongue, open your eyes wide, and cross them to look at your nose. Exhale with a loud *haaaaa*. Release down, head into your hands and rock your hips.

7 Locust

Salabhasana

Lift your legs, arms, and head off the floor with arms extended fully in front of you. Hold three to five breaths. Release to the floor, head in your hands, and rock your hips side to side.

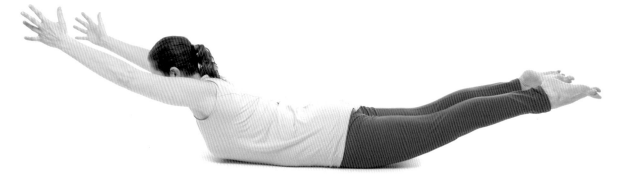

8   Bow with Kidney 1 Pulse

Dhanurasana

Lie on your belly and bend both knees so your feet come toward your butt. Reach around and hold on to your ankles. If you can't reach, use a strap wrapped around both your ankles. If you can easily reach your feet, try holding your feet so your thumbs are pressing into Kidney 1 (the hollow between the ball of your first and second toes). Hold here deeply as you press your feet away from your butt, opening up into the pose. Hold three to five breaths and slowly lower down, releasing your head to your hands. Rock your hips. Repeat two more times.

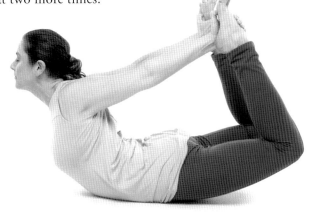

9   Child's Pose

Balasana

Press back into child's pose for five breaths. Stack your hands and rest your head on your hands.

10   Plank to Dog Flow

Press back into downward dog and hold several breaths. Come forward to plank pose and hold several breaths. Go back and forth between these two poses five times, holding each pose for three to five breaths.

11   Snake Dog

Hold downward dog for five to ten breaths, moving your spine, hips, and shoulders in any way that feels good, opening, and undulating your spine. See the online video.

12   Hang

Uttanasana

Walk your feet in to your hands and hang in a full forward bend for several breaths.

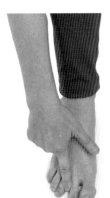
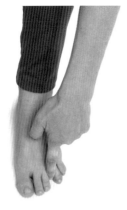

13   Squat with Gate Clear

Bend your knees and come into a squat, using padding under your heels, if you need, to stabilize the pose. Clear the gates on your hands and feet (see instructions on page 80). Come into a hang to release for several breaths. Slowly roll back up to stand.

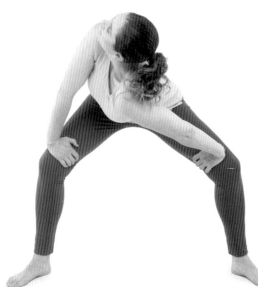

14   Horse with Crossover Stretch

Separate your feet three feet apart, turn your toes out slightly, and bend your knees. Rest your hands on your thighs, fingers pointing down. Cross one shoulder over the centerline of your body and turn your body upward, looking up. Breathe deeply for three to five breaths. Switch sides. Do both sides again.

15   Flapping the Abdominal Wall

Uddiyana Bandha Kriya

Note: Do not do this if you are on your menstrual cycle or are pregnant.

Stay in the same position as the prior pose and exhale all the air out of your belly. Hold the exhale out, apply mula bandha, and jalandhara bandha, and flap the abdominal wall in and out, pulling your belly in and pushing it out. When you need to inhale again, release the held breath and the bandhas and then slowly inhale coming to stand. Do the whole sequence again. (This *kriya*, an action designed to have a specific outcome, has different names in different yoga traditions.) See the online video.

16 Aura Fluff Out, Fluff In

Come back to standing and bring your feet closer together. Sweep one arm out and up overhead, and then draw your hand consciously down the centerline of your body. Do this several times on both sides. Now reverse the motion. Starting at the bottom of the centerline of your body, sweep your hand up the centerline of your body, out, and down. Do this several times on both sides. See the online video.

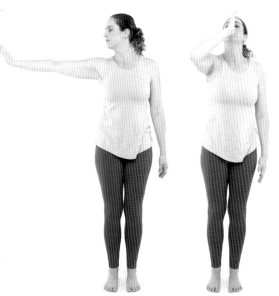

17 Standing Backbend

Stand in tadasana and lift your heart center up into a gentle backbend with your hands in Triple Warmer/Heart mudra. Hold three to five breaths without straining. Engage your low back and upper abdominal muscles to support the pose. Try to keep tension out of your neck. You can use jalandara bandha to help.

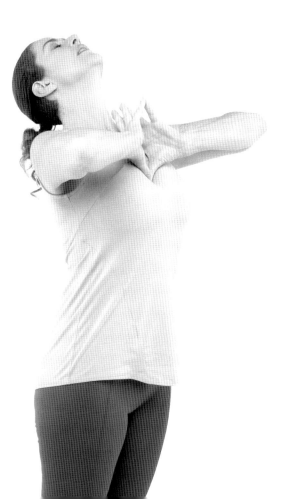

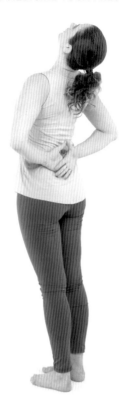

18 Standing Backbend with Ming Man Point Rub

Standing in tadasana, lift your heart center up into a gentle backbend. You can go a bit deeper this time, including lifting your chin up, as long as there is no strain. Bring your hands to your low back and make circles directly behind your belly button, which is the Ming Man point. This point is called the "Sea of Vitality" and is used for longevity and overall strength.

19 Heaven Rushing In

Release your hands up overhead as you continue your backbend. Arms are open in a V, with palms facing the sky. Hold here several breaths, allowing energy, inspiration, and joy to fill you. Come back to tadasana. Bring one hand over the other on top of your heart center.

20 Hug and Massage/Free Shoulder Blades (Wings)

Give yourself a big hug around your shoulder blades. If possible, press your fingers deeply in and massage under the edges of your shoulder blades, releasing the fascia.

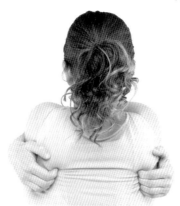

21 King Dancer with Meridian Finger Press and Lion Face

Natarajasana

Stand strongly on your right leg, lift and bend your left leg behind you, and reach around with your left arm to hold your ankle or foot. You can use a strap around your ankle if you can't reach your foot. If you can, press your thumb deeply into Kidney 1 as you start to pull your foot away from your body. Reach your right hand out and press your thumb against each finger until you find the one that feels like it's offering you the most stability to the pose. Press your thumb strongly to that finger as you continue developing the pose, lifting your heart center and opening your left foot away from your body. Breathe here for five to seven breaths.

On your last two breaths, stick out your tongue, cross your eyes if you can, and exhale with an audible *haaaaa*. Then slowly release the pose. Repeat on the other side.

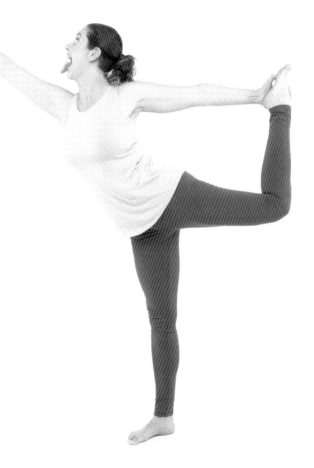

22 EMYoga-Haka

Separate your feet about the width of your mat and turn out your toes slightly. With strong force, pound your fists against your chest two times, and then open them up fully and face them forward (jazz hands). At the same time, make a lion's face and roar: tongue out, eyes crossed, audible roaring exhale. Repeat this three times. (Haka is the traditional war cry/dance of the Maori first peoples of New Zealand—with deepest respect to the people from the "land of the long white cloud," where my spiritual path began.) See the online video.

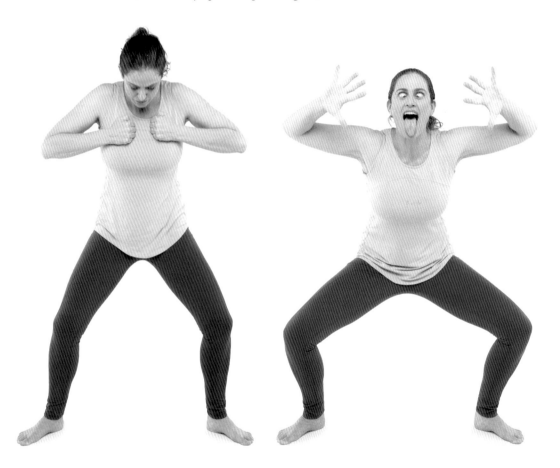

23 Bringing Down the Flame

See complete instructions on
page 88 and the online video.

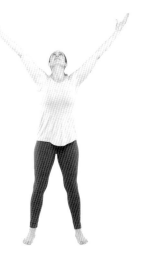

24 Handstand Against Wall or Handstand Prep, Inverted L Against Wall

Adho Mukha Vriksasana

Come to the wall and take downward dog with your hands six to eight inches
from the wall. Walk your feet in, and with your left knee bent, jump your
right leg up toward the wall. It might take several tries before you manage
to stay inverted. Hold here several breaths, and then come down and rest in
child's pose. Do the pose again, jumping with your other leg.

   Alternatively, do downward dog with your heels against the wall. Slowly walk
your legs up the wall until you are in the shape of an inverted L. You may need
to come down to adjust your arm position so that your shoulders are directly
over your wrists. Hold several breaths and then release into child's pose.

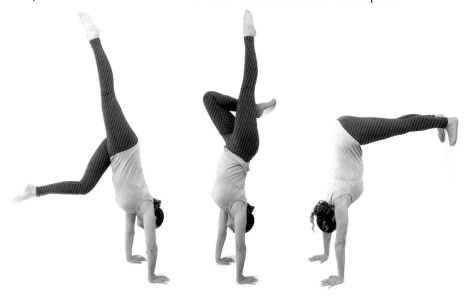

25 Slow Sit-Ups with Hook Up

Do five sit-ups with no momentum or pulling. (See page 92 for instructions and the online video.)

26 Moving Bridge with Fire Neurolymphatic Clear

Dwi Pada Pitham

Inhale and lift up into bridge with arms overhead. Exhale and release down. Do this five times. Come up again and hold the pose for five breaths, then release. (See instructions on page 94.)

While resting, massage the points shown. To massage strongly under the last rib, you have to relax deeply, and then you can actually slip your fingers up and under the bone. This might feel strange, but stay with it. Massage along the entire bone. When you're done, you can lift up again into bridge and exhale with a few audible *haaaaa* sounds.

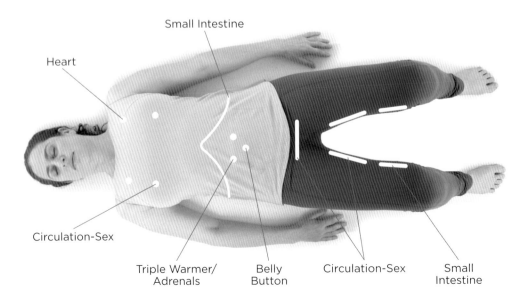

Small Intestine

Heart

Circulation-Sex

Triple Warmer/ Adrenals

Belly Button

Circulation-Sex

Small Intestine

27 Fish with Chakra Clear

Matsyasana
See full instructions on page 97
and the online video.

Note: If you are used to releasing
your hands from the floor in fish
pose, you can clear the chakra
channels while up in the full pose.

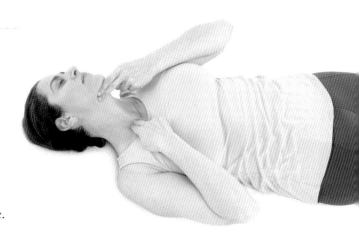

28 Triple Warmer Sedate and Control on Back

Lie on your back and cross your right leg over your left bent knee. Draw your
left knee in toward your chest. Hold around the outside of your left calf, just
below your knee (Stomach 36). Wrap your right hand around your left elbow
(Triple Warmer 10). Hold for two minutes. Switch sides.

To hold the control points for Triple Warmer, cross your feet at your ankles
with your right foot closest to your body. Wrap your left hand around the
outside of your left foot on the edge of your pinky toe (Bladder 66). Take your
right hand and hold it at the junction between your pinky and ring finger of
your left hand (Triple Warmer 2), as shown below. Hold for one minute and
switch sides.

Alternatively, you can do
the pose as outlined in the
water practice on page 112.

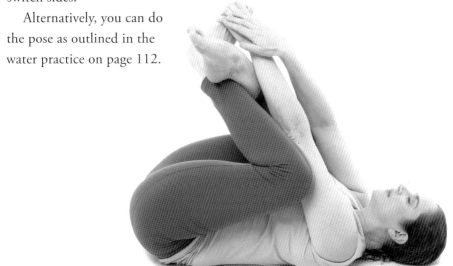

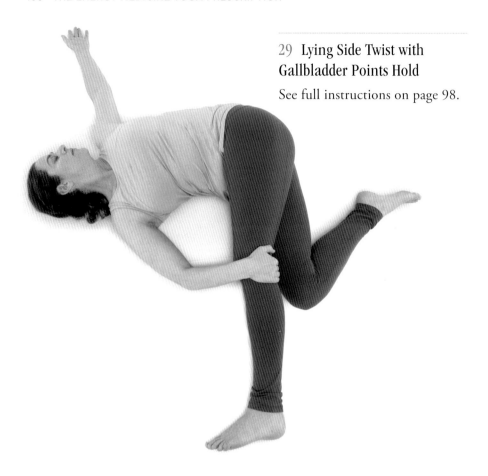

29 Lying Side Twist with Gallbladder Points Hold

See full instructions on page 98.

30 Savasana Prep with Fire Neurovascular Reflex Points Hold

Bring one hand to cover your forehead. Bring your other hand to hold directly behind your eyes on the back of your skull. Hold here for one to two minutes. Exhale several times with a *haaaaa*, then release into full savasana.

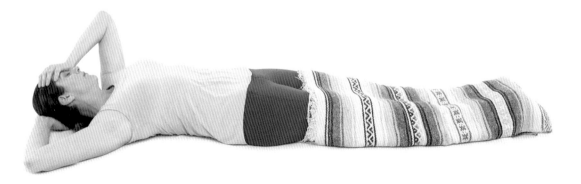

31 Savasana

Completely surrender and relax for five to fifteen minutes.

32 Pranayama: Kapalabhati

Note: Do not do this pranayama sequence if you are on your menstrual cycle or pregnant.

Sit comfortably with your spine straight. This pranayama uses a sharp exhalation from the nose, followed by a natural inhalation. The focus is on the exhalation, letting the breath come back in naturally. It is similar to blowing your nose, and in fact, you might want some tissues handy. Start with a full deep inhale and a full deep exhale. Then take a comfortable inhale and begin: sharp exhalation, followed by natural inhalation. Do one round of nine, then pause and take a full deep inhale and exhale. Next round, do eighteen. Next round, do twenty-seven. See the online video.

33 Meditation

The fire meditation is called Fire in Belly: a meditation on the navel. Come to a comfortable seat, with your spine straight. Bring your awareness to your navel center. Visualize a golden flame in your navel. Sit for five to twenty minutes. When you are complete, place one finger in your belly button and one finger at your third eye. With both fingers, push in and pull slightly up as you inhale through your nose and exhale out your mouth three times.

ADDITIONAL FIRE PRACTICE FOR INSOMNIA:
Brazilian Toe Technique

Sleep is one of the three pillars of health, so getting a good night sleep consistently is incredibly important to health and healing.

It doesn't matter when in the day you do this technique; it helps you fall asleep when it's time to. I've also done this in bed in the middle of the night when I've woken up and can't get back to sleep. Then I just fold one leg up and do one at a time so I can remain lying down.

In EMYoga we do this toward the end of the practice. If you can sit in full lotus, do so. You can also do this in a simple cross-legged position. It's helpful if you can reach both feet at the same time, but if not, you can do one at a time—it'll just take you longer. See the online video of the Brazilian Toe Technique.

For our purposes, we'll number the toes one through five, starting with one as the big toe and five as the little (pinky) toe. Similarly, we'll number the fingers one through five, starting with the thumb as number one and the pinky finger as number five. You can do either one foot at a time or both together. It works best if you use the opposite hand to foot.

Bring your third finger to your third toe covering the toenail. Slide your thumb under your third toe. Hold two to three minutes with a light touch. Keeping some form of contact, slide your thumb under your fourth toe and move your fourth finger onto the toenail of your fourth toe. Hold two to three minutes. Slide your thumb under your pinky toe, and put your pinky finger on the toenail of your pinky toe. Hold two to three minutes. Next, slide your thumb under your second toe. Put your index finger on the second toenail. Hold two to three minutes. Then slide your thumb under your big toe. Place your index and middle finger on the toenail of your big toe. Hold two to three minutes.

Sweet dreams . . .

Earth

Earth is all about relationships—our relationship to ourselves, our relationship to everyone else in our lives, as well as our relationship to our environment, our pets, and our jobs. It encompasses the meridians of Spleen and Stomach. Spleen is about upward-moving energy, the energy that keeps our organs from prolapsing, which could not be more important, especially as we age. Spleen is also the nurturing part of the immune system. It governs the blood, the very life force of the body. Stomach is about self-love. We can see that in a very literal way in how we are lovingly nourished by food. It can also be seen in how often food is abused in our lives. Many of us have succumbed to the pint of ice cream or the entire pizza on the couch when licking our wounds from some kind of hurt. Those "comfort" foods act as a substitute for the real love and nourishment we didn't get. Stomach is a yang meridian, but it's the only yang meridian that runs on the yin (front) side of the body. This shows us the need to bring an internal, comforting nature into this outward, active energy in order to be fully fed and nourished with the sweetness of self-regard.

The Psychology of Earth

Earth people are the ones who are the natural caretakers. They are the first ones to volunteer to help in any event or circumstance, regardless of how much they already have on their plate. They are the ones serving in the soup kitchen, baking the cookies for the school fundraiser, answering phones during the political campaign. They can also be the busy bodies, sticking their two cents into everyone else's business, offering advice and council, whether asked for or not.

On the flip side of this, when earth people are out of balance, they can be the very ones ignoring their own needs. They take care of everyone except themselves. Boundaries are their issue, and they can often get taken advantage of because they are so giving. They can also wear themselves out because of lack of self-care. They need to turn the focus around from pointing outwardly to pointing inwardly. They need to care as much for their own well-being as they do for everyone else's. This is the idea of "right relationship"—the ability to discern how to be with others and the strength to implement that. Out-of-balance earth can also show up as greed or disregard for the rest of the tribe or community. You see that with people who are lazy, who take the biggest piece of pie first before anyone else is served. You see it writ large as our corporations and the biggest wealth holders on the planet hoard resources far in excess of what they could ever consume—a hedge against an underlying fear of loss and lack of love. It is classic Freudian pathology. But who is going to tell the Koch brothers that their unholy greed and destruction of Earth herself is because they do not have enough self-love? It is a difficult conversation to have, but really, the healing of the planet comes down to that, the healing of the individuals who are on the planet. We are living in an Earth-imbalanced time, and we will survive only if we learn to love the very thing we are destroying.

The history of the Five Elements can also help us understand how we've gotten to this place and how to move forward into a place of healing and care, both for ourselves and our planet. Originally the Five Elements were the four elements: earth was in the center, and water, wood, fire, and metal surrounded it. Sara Allen, advanced EM practitioner and one of the founding faculty members of Innersource, writes: "Earth was seen as the only and original regulator in the body . . . and damage to Stomach or Spleen—the taproots of the body—damaged the entire assimilation and movement of chi. When Stomach and Spleen were damaged, the roots of the body were damaged, making sustenance on Earth either a quick or a slow deterioration."[1]

The four-element design makes a lot of sense if you look at the elements as seasons. Each season has a midpoint—the summer and winter solstices and the spring and autumn equinoxes—that are the technical starting points of the seasons as well as the height of those seasons. Each season would wind its way back into the center, then back out for its duration, into the center to transition, and back out to complete its cycle. There is a beautiful elegance to this pattern and a perfect balance to the four points. We always return to the center for balance, and Earth, our very home, is the place from which all the elements arise.

In the old system, with the earth element in the center, Spleen and Stomach were more involved in each of the other seasons. They are the carriers of nourishment, love, self-care, and grounding. As we cycled around the wheel, every midpoint would bring us back to this emphasis on our connection to the earth and the emphasis on the compassion that we need to move forward in our lives. At this point, too, Triple Warmer and Circulation-Sex, the two meridians in charge of circulating energy and nourishment to every other system in the body, were in service to Spleen and Stomach. They followed them around the wheel, doing the bidding of the earth element. Sara Allen reminds us, "Triple Warmer is all about external protection; Circulation-Sex is all about internal protection. They're both systems of protection."[2] Triple Warmer and Circulation-Sex supported Spleen and Stomach so they could fully nourish the body, offering internal and external protection as we went through our cycles.

Earth was moved out of the center of the wheel in China (approximately 1100 BC) around the same time that the European world was moving away from a partnership society toward a more masculine-dominated war-centric society.[3] With this change in the wheel, Spleen and Stomach moved to the outside, and so did their helpers. Triple Warmer and Circulation-Sex were elevated to their own element, fire. Earth, then, became just one of the Five Elements, its status diminished and put on the same level as the other four elements.

Now, before we relegate earth back to the center, it's important to look at both the benefits and the deficits of the system of four versus five. With earth in the center and the four other elements radiating out, it is balanced yet static. There is no movement between the elements in terms of a continual, modifying influence. With earth moved to the outside, becoming the fifth element, there is a dynamic flow of energy between all the elements, both around the outside ring (the flow cycle) and by creating the star inside (the control cycle). This more accurately expresses how energy flows around and through the body and gives us a very powerful working map for how to increase that flow, jump-start it, and direct it when energy gets stuck.

What we really want is yet another example of both-and. We want to elevate earth back into the center of our lives at the same time as keeping the dynamic movement of the Five Elements alive. This isn't just metaphorical. We need only look at the rampant destruction of Earth herself in our world to see how out of balance we are with Triple Warmer, the masculine, controlling force in dominance. It is obvious that we cannot continue this way, and that we simply will not survive at all if we destroy the very substance on which we rely for every aspect of life. If we elevate earth to the center again, we can begin the long path toward mending the damage we've done, both on Earth herself and on the earth within ourselves. And keeping the Five Element Wheel as it currently is, we have this powerful map for affecting all areas of our lives, depending on the needs of the moment. We need to be more loving, more caring, more compassionate with ourselves and with others, and we need to do the same with the planet.

The Physiology of Earth

The poses that help balance earth are forward bends and twists; these poses help enormously with digestion and elimination. Seated forward bends, when you're relying on the earth to support you, allow you to turn your focus deeply inward. Interestingly, the sound for earth is the sound of the ujjayi breath. This is the main breath used in all yoga asana practices, and it is telling that this is the breath that helps heal the divide between caring too much for others and not enough for the self.

We also bring in the sedating of Circulation-Sex here, not in the fire practice. The reason is explained by Sara Allen: "When we support Circulation-Sex, we strengthen Spleen. Spleen is responsible for feeding the organs. Circulation-Sex is the intelligence that equitably distributes what Spleen has to offer. Stomach energy, the Circulation-Sex yang partner, brings the chi in; Spleen digests and assimilates it; and Circulation-Sex allocates according to essential needs of the rhythms of the organs."[4]

The movement here that helps propel earth into the next element of metal is the inward loop, spiraling in to spiral out, like a snail burrowing inside to expand outward to its next life.

Earth Properties

Governs	Blood
Season	Solstice/Equinox
Meridians	Spleen (yin), Stomach (yang)
Archetypes	The Earth mother, the peacemaker
Main Emotions	Challenging: Overcompassion for others, worry Balancing: Self-love

The EMYoga Earth Practice

1 Wake Up

Do the Wake Up seated, and use a gentle touch, tapping lightly or massaging. Earth is the element of self-love, so it's important during this practice to be kind to your body, substituting the powerful thumping for a gentle rhythm. See page 78 for instructions and the online video.

2 Pranayama

Practice ujjayi pranayama at the start to set your breath for the entire sequence. See instructions on page 69.

3 Spleen and Stomach Meridian Clear

Massage deeply along the Spleen and Stomach lines as shown. The Spleen meridian starts at the big toe and moves up. The Stomach meridian starts under the eye and moves down.

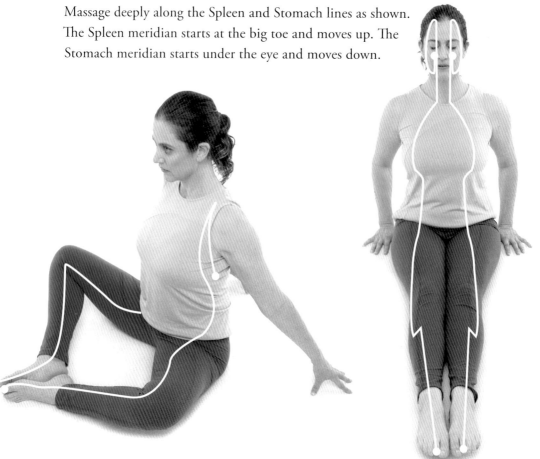

4 Circulation-Sex Sedate and Control in Starfish

From seated, bring your feet to the floor with legs bent, and flop them both over to the right, but separated and offset from each other so that the inner edge of your left leg and the outer edge of your right leg are on the floor. Bring your right hand to the edge of the ball of your right foot and place your fingers on the downhill slope (Spleen 3). Place your left fingertips under the right wrist crease in the exact center of your right wrist (Circulation-Sex 7). Hold here two to three minutes. While you're holding, play around with the opening or sensation you're feeling in your hips. Then simply flop your legs over to the other side and hold the same points here for two to three minutes.

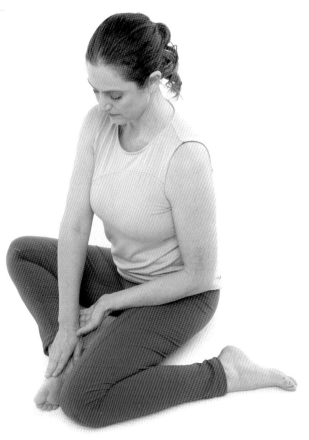

Hold the Control Points
Stay on this side with your legs to the left, and slide your left thumb into the left bent knee crease, directly over the thick ropy tendon you can feel (Kidney 10). With your right hand, hold in the exact center of the elbow crease of your left arm (Circulation-Sex 3). Hold for one minute. Then flop your legs over to the right and hold this second set of points there.

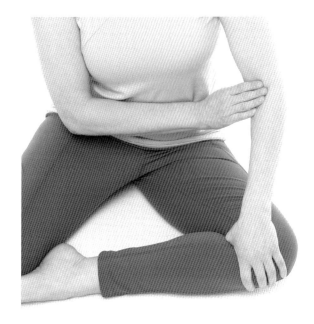

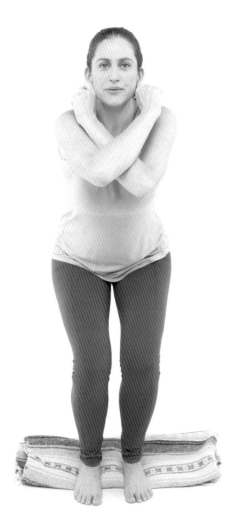

5 Squat to Stand

Note: Do not do this pose if you're pregnant or menstruating.

Come into a squat (with supportive padding if you need it). Cross your hands in front of your body, with your right hand in front, and hold on to your opposite earlobes. Have your thumbs on the front and your fingers on the back of your earlobes. Bring your tongue to the roof of your mouth. Inhale and slowly come up to stand. Exhale out the mouth. Now inhale as you go down and exhale out the mouth as you rise up. Do this several times, inhaling on the way down and exhaling, out the mouth, on the way up. Also try this breathing in and out of the nose. Eventually build up to twelve to fourteen squats. You don't need to come all the way down to a full squat every time.[5] See the online video.

6 Squat Lunge

From a squat, remove the padding and use your hands for support on the floor in front of the body. Staying as low in the squat as possible, thrust your right leg back into a squat lunge. Breathe here a couple of breaths, and then bring your right leg back and thrust out your left leg. Your goal here is to try to stay low in the squat while coming into a lunge. Do three each side.

7   Long Hang with Gate Clear

Uttanasana

Release your hips up to the air, head down to the earth. Hook your arms elbow to elbow and allow yourself to release. Allow an ample bend in your knee. Stay here five to ten breaths. Then release your arms and clear the gates on your hands (see page 80 for gate clearing instructions).

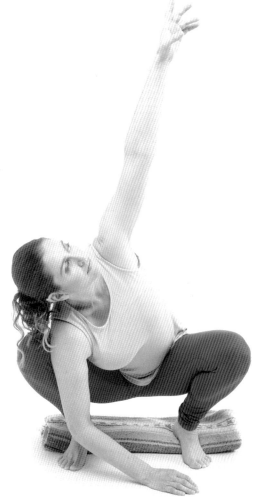

8   Squat with Twist

Come back down to the squat with padding. Bring your right arm between your legs, rest your palm on the floor, and lift your left arm up, coming into a twist. Flick your fingers one at a time against your thumb. Circle your left wrist several times, and when you're ready to release, smooth your hand back and forth through your aura, in a figure eight pattern, until you bring that arm between your legs and twist to the other side, repeating the hand movements.

9 Downward Dog with Leg-Under Twist

Adho Mukha Svanasana

Step back to downward dog, and take several breaths here, loosening up your legs, spine, shoulders, and neck. Now lift your right leg up into the air behind you, keeping your hips aligned at first. Take a few breaths and then open up your hip as wide as feels good, but keeping your shoulders squared. Then draw your leg forward and turn your hips to bring your leg under your torso to the left, sliding your leg along the ground and lowering your body until you're in a forward lying-down twist. Turn your head in whichever direction feels the most comfortable. Hold three to five breaths, and slowly uncurl yourself. Come back to downward dog for a few regulating breaths, including a rest for a few breaths in child's pose. Repeat on the other side. Then walk your feet in to your hands, hang over for several breaths, and roll up, tracing Spleen.

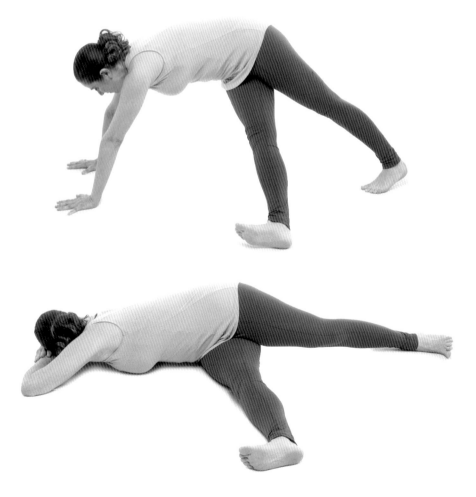

10 Belt Flow with Spleen Up

Bring both hands to your right waist as far as possible, even slightly around to the back. Press in firmly and smooth both hands around to your left waist. Release your hands and go back to your far right waist. Again, pull deeply and firmly across your belly to your left waist. Do this one more time. At the last arrival to your left waist, smooth your hands down the outside of your left leg and off your pinky toe. Hang over for a moment, then come up tracing Spleen (see page 81). Repeat on the other side. See the online video.

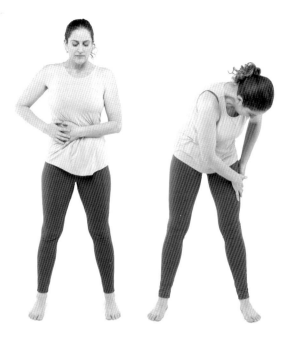

11 Ileocecal/Houston Valve Clear

Straighten your legs to stand with your feet slightly more than hip-width apart, and bring your hands flat over your low belly, with your pinky fingers on the crest of your hip bone. Inhale and press your fingers deeply into your belly and pull up. Exhale and shake off your hands. Bring your hands to the same position and do it again. Inhale, pressing deeply in and pulling up. Do it one more time. Now bring your hands to your low ribs, inhale, and on your exhale, press your fingers deeply in and smooth down. Shake off your hands. See the online video.

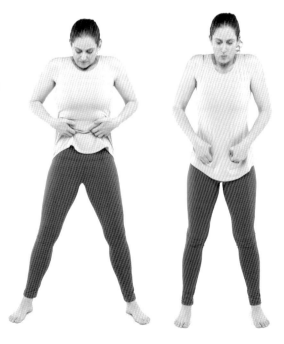

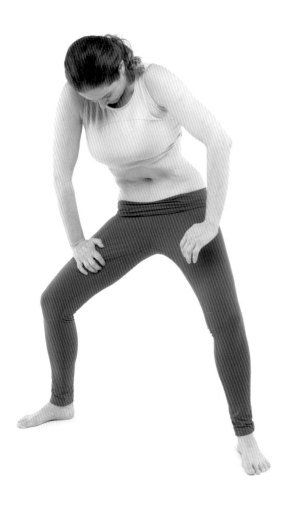

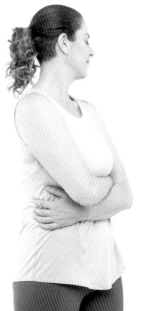

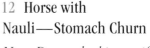

12 Horse with Nauli—Stomach Churn

Note: Do not do this pose if you're pregnant or menstruating.

Step your feet apart two to three feet and turn your toes slightly out. Support your upper body with your hands on your thighs. Exhale all your breath out. Hold your breath out, and draw your belly in toward your spine as powerfully as you can. At the same time draw in mula bandha and tip your chin toward your chest for jalandhara bandha. Continue holding your breath out, and walk your hands back and forth on your legs, exchanging the full weight of your body from hand to hand, from side to side. This is the start of doing the full nauli, stomach churning. Eventually you can move your belly cavity this way without the use of your hands. When you need to inhale again, stop the motion, release the belly pull, and inhale. See the online video.

13 Cradling the Baby

See complete instructions on page 90 and the online video.

14 Triangle with Spleen-Liver-Kidney (SLK) Point Clear

Trikonasana

Step your left foot back two to three feet and turn your toes out forty-five degrees. Turn your body to the side. Bring your arms out to the sides and tilt over at your waist, bringing your right hand down to your right calf.

Note: Do not do the SLK Point Clear if you are pregnant. Find the SLK point—the junction of Spleen, Liver, and Kidney—on your inner right calf (about a hand's span up from the center inner face of your Achilles tendon). You'll know when you find the point because it'll feel like a slight dip inward and will most likely be painful when you press deeply. If you can't reach the SLK point in triangle, just rest your lower hand lightly wherever it lands on your leg. Massage here deeply with your thumb, and then maintain the pose with your thumb pressing this spot, but without resting your body weight on your arm. Use the strength of your legs to support you. Stay three to five breaths. Inhale, activating your legs and the side body to bring yourself back up to stand. Repeat on the other side or do the next two poses in sequence as a short flow.

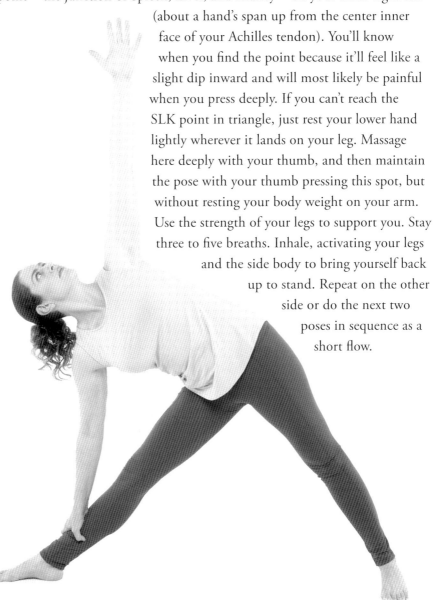

15 Twisting Triangle

Parivrtta Trikonasana

From triangle with your right leg forward, turn your back toes slightly more forward and perhaps step your back foot a bit closer to the front. Inhale and bring your arms out to the sides. Twist from the waist, and bring your left arm forward, right arm up. Bring your left arm to the outside of your right leg, deepening the twist. Bring your hand to wherever you can reach on your right leg. You can press in anywhere on the outward right calf, massaging down toward your foot on what is the Stomach line, the calf portion of the Stomach meridian. Then rest your hand on the floor or your calf and take three to five deep breaths.

16 Twisting Half-Moon

Parivrtta Ardha Chandrasana

If you feel comfortable in twisting triangle, from there you can lift your left leg off the floor, coming into twisting half-moon. You might want to have a block under your left hand to help stabilize the pose. Open up your right arm toward the sky. Hold here three to five breaths. Then slowly lower down to a squat for a few breaths, and repeat the entire sequence (of three poses) on the other side.

17 Pigeon with Rooster Comb Hold

Eka Pada Rajakapotasana

Come into downward dog, and step your right knee forward between your hands and lower down. If you find your hips dropping to the right side, put a folded blanket under your right hip to bring your hips into balance.

First, use your hands, pressing into the floor, to help you lift and open your back, in a gentle backbend. Then slowly lower down as much as you can. Depending on how far to the floor you are, you'll either prop your arms on a block or bolster to do the Rooster Comb Hold. If you can't release your hands from the floor at all in this pose, simply come into starfish. If you're lying all the way or close to the ground, turn your head to the left (this is a personal preference—if it feels better to turn toward your knee, do that). Bring the heel of one hand to your forehead and drape your hand over the top of your head so your fingers are on the crown. Place the heel of your other hand where the top of your head starts to curve back, and drape those fingers also over the crown until they meet the other fingers at the top of your head. You can modify this hand hold any way that works for you as long as you're covering the centerline of your head, from your forehead, over the top, to the back of your head behind your forehead. Stay here two to five minutes. Repeat on the other side.

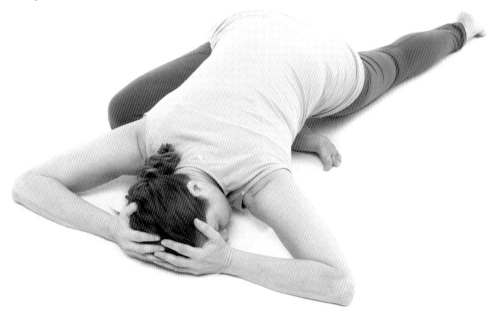

18 Moving Bridge with Earth Neurolymphatic Clear

Dwi Pada Pitham

Lie on your back with your feet bent about a foot from your butt. Lift your hips up and your arms up overhead on inhale; exhale hips down, arms down. Repeat three to five times. Then hold up in the lifted pose three to five breaths. Release down, and let your knees gently rest against each other. Massage the points as shown.

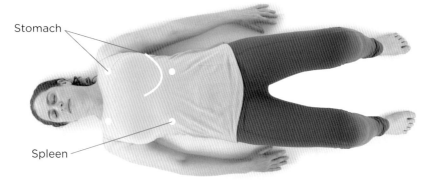

Stomach

Spleen

19 Spleen Strengthen

Janusirsasana

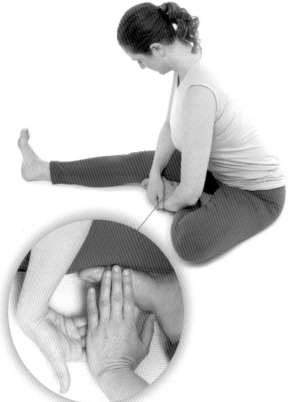

From seated, straighten your right leg and bend your left leg, placing your foot against your inner right thigh in janusirsasana. With your left hand, hold the points on the uphill slope of the edge of the ball of your foot (Spleen 2). Wrap your right hand around the pinky-side edge of your left hand to cover the front of your palm in line with your little finger (Heart 8). Hold two to three minutes. At the same time, continue to deepen the pose, bending from your hips. Inhale, tracing up Spleen to release from the pose, and switch sides. *Note:* If you're very flexible, you can hold these points on the extended right leg. See *Energy Medicine Yoga* for picture reference.

20 Spleen Control in Seated Forward Bend

Paschimottanasana

If you can easily reach your toes with your legs extended out in front of you, hold the control points here. Otherwise, bring the soles of your feet together, knees apart, in baddha konasana. Either way, bring the first two fingers from each hand to cover the base of your big toe toenail (Spleen 1 and Liver 1). Bend forward from your hips and hold for one minute.

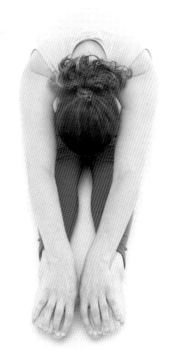

21 Inclined Plane or Tabletop

Purvottanasana

Rise up from paschimottanasana and bring your hands by your hips, fingertips pointing toward your toes. Inhale and lift your body off the floor in one straight plane (purvottanasana). You can also do tabletop if that feels better for your body. Hold here, breathing deeply for five to ten breaths. Alternately, you can do breath of fire, rapid inhalations and exhalations through your nose for thirty seconds to one minute.

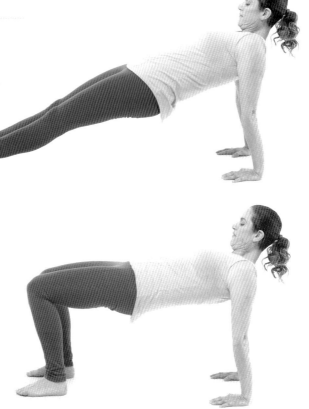

22   Savasana Prep with Earth Neurovascular Reflex Points Hold

Lie on your back with your legs rolled open, relaxed. Bring your palms over your eye sockets with the heels of your hands resting on the cheekbones. Stay here until you feel yourself starting to deeply relax. Then bring your arms to your side body, palms facing up.

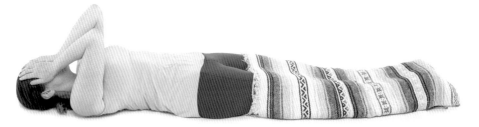

23   Savasana

Rest in savasana for five to fifteen minutes.

24   Meditation

Come to a comfortable seat with your spine straight. Take several smooth, deep inhales, then simply relax and let your body settle. Bring your awareness to your root chakra, at the base of your spine. Visualize roots coming out from your body and sinking into the earth. Allow yourself to feel not only grounded but also connected to the earth through these tendrils of roots that run from your body deep into the ground and spread wide all around you. These roots, like the roots of the trees, are interconnected with the roots of everyone on the planet. Feel this connection as the quiet, underground whispering of the microbes and mycelium that interconnect the unseen world. Allow this feeling of connection to filter back up from the roots, into your body. Rise up this feeling of connection, through your spine, directly into your heart chakra. Feel the beating of your heart in rhythm with the pulse of the earth. Bring both hands to rest, one on top of the other, over the heart chakra. As you hold your heart, let this energy continue to rise up and out your crown, connecting you with the heavens and the pure potential. Repeat the bija mantra "lam" (pronounced lum), the sound for earth energy, several times, either silently or out loud. End your meditation with one audible *lam*.

ADDITIONAL EARTH PRACTICE:
EMYoga and Your Menstrual Cycle

One of the debates women have within the yoga tradition is whether to practice during their menstrual cycle. The general consensus is that women should not do inversions during this time, as they can lead to problems such as endometriosis. This is because blood is trying to leave the body flowing downward, and you turn that upside down when you practice, going against the natural flow. Other than that, there is very little guidance for women during this time.

Most women look at the menstrual cycle as a nuisance at best and a curse at worst. The culture at large has also taken a stance on this, determining that women are unfit for certain responsibilities because they are "irrational" once a month. Most religions consider women "unclean" and keep them from performing any religious rites as a result of this. Dr. John Douillard, noted Ayurvedic physician, writes in his book *Body, Mind & Sport* that in our culture, many women "regard this time as no different from any other time of the month, and as a result they experience only the problems, and not the benefits of menstruation."[6]

A woman's menstrual cycle is a mechanism for cleansing the body. There is some science that says this cleansing process is one of the reasons women live longer than men. But many women suffer PMS, cramps, and pain, which are generally caused by hormonal and energetic imbalances. These can often be mitigated by both energetic and Ayurvedic means.

Donna Eden suffered strongly from the hormonal disturbances of PMS. She writes eloquently in her book *Energy Medicine for Women* that there is a powerful connection with our own innermost guides during the menstrual cycle that is not available to the other gender, and she suggests we could learn how to celebrate it: "PMS is nature's design for making you reexamine your life intensively for a few days every month."[7] There are other positive aspects to PMS, Donna writes: "PMS potentially holds a positive, creative, rehabilitative function. Like the sacred plants used in shamanic healing ceremonies to open a doorway to the world of spirit, PMS changes the body's chemistry to clear a path for consciously journeying into the domain of the soul."[8]

Many women I've spoken with say they suffer cramps or discomfort and that practicing yoga or doing some other form of physical exercise is the only thing that relieves them of these monthly pains. Douillard addresses this beautifully in his book: "If the prana, or vital energy, needed to maintain normal menstrual functioning is siphoned off to support the energy needs of exercise or work, ultimately it will lead to imbalance and the body's inability to menstruate efficiently. The reproductive organs, weakened by overtraining during the menstrual period, will drain the body's energy reserve, creating the classic PMS symptoms."[9] He elaborates further on why women feel temporary relief during their periods by exercising:

> Exercise can force the body to adapt and compensate, to take much-needed energy from the reproductive organs in order to produce a temporary sense of well-being. This can only leave the body in a more depleted condition, susceptible to future menstrual difficulties. Many healthy women can get away with not taking extra rest during their menstrual flow. In the short run, they will be symptom-free. But from a preventive point of view, for later in life during and after menopause, give your body the chance to take rest if it needs it.[10]

This does not mean that women must simply suffer through three to five days a month. But what it does point to is a deeper need to listen to the body, to tune in and take stock. For many women, it isn't possible to take the first three days of their period as vacation days. But for most of us, it is possible to lessen the load.

I concede that it isn't easy stopping the momentum of life. Whether you have the luxury of taking a day or two off when your moon begins, or you work full time and can't simply call in sick two days a month, doesn't seem to matter. For some women, the intensity of the menstrual cycle literally forces them to take time out of their regular lives, and I submit that this is a biological imperative that has developed in our too busy world to enforce a mind-set that nature designed.

When a woman's cycle is being used against her, in such fields as religion, politics, and commerce, it is often said that she can't think clearly during this time because her body and mind are flooded with hormones, and therefore she is ill-equipped to make important decisions in the heat of the moment, which could come at any time. This is where the overwhelming patriarchy has it entirely wrong. This time of a woman's cycle every month is destined to keep everything in balance, and the leaders of the world, women included (who are still leading in the template designed by men, instead of leading from a woman's perspective), should take note of this instead of dismissing it as untenable. The truth is, the world could use a little more perspective and careful, thoughtful, compassionate analyses, instead of rash, judgmental, unstoppable forward momentum without checks on speed, force, or rightness of the decisions.

The most power a woman has at her disposal is the ability to stop, turn inward, and check over all the decisions and actions she's made in the previous month to review for their accuracy and grace. It is a time when a woman has deeper access to her intuition, to the frequencies of truth that are constantly resonating all around us if we just got quiet enough to listen.

I'm writing this with the hope that women start to practice this. If enough of us hold that space, then the morphic field strengthens, and more and more women will be drawn into the field of feeling empowered and gifted with our natural processes.

If you can, or if you are willing, or if you simply want to, try this: the next first day of your moon, do absolutely nothing. No exercise. No work. No chores. Sleep late. Take a bath. Drink tea in your bathrobe. Sit in the window seat and watch the sky. Walk slowly around the garden, in the snow, or in the grass. Don't get anywhere, just amble. Look at things. Be a child. Let the world fascinate you. Let the world sadden you. Let the world inspire you and ignite you. Let yourself be, with no judgment or agenda.

The day will feel endless. Let it. You will feel bored at points. Let yourself. You might feel emotions run, course, rage, spill through your body. Let them. Let it all be. Just let yourself be. For one day a month. Let nothing at all happen.

If it's possible, do very little on the next two days. If you must work, work. But don't add extra things to your day. Don't exercise. Don't socialize. Just be as quiet and as planning-less as possible. If you don't have the luxury to take a complete day off, try to lessen your load. Ask others to help with your daily responsibilities. If you must be at work, see if you can go slower, take a few extra breaks, and don't do anything that isn't essential. Refrain from exercising, and if possible, rest more.

When you come back from this reflective time, notice how you feel. Notice if the decisions you made last week, before you took this time off, still stand. Did you make the right choice? Are there places in your life you need to be more fierce? Stand up for yourself or others? Be assertive? Are there places in your life you need to soften more? To listen deeper? To have more compassion, forgiveness?

Imagine if the whole world did this, if men did this too, if, before we went rushing headlong into a war, we thought, we pulled back, we retreated, we consulted with our deepest inner knowing. Imagine what the world might be like.

We create our world. Each of us, by our own actions, and collectively, by what we teach and share and show each other. We can re-create our world at any moment. We just have to take the first step forward. And sometimes that step forward is a step inward.

In terms of a yoga practice, my recommendations are to refrain from practicing any form of asana during the first three days of your cycle. Other practices that you can do are free-form meditation, alternate nostril breathing, and savasana. Also, in EMYoga, thankfully guided by the challenges that Donna faced, we have tools to help mitigate the extreme discomfort and bring the body back into hormonal balance so we don't suffer so much physical pain.

If you suffer from PMS, add in the following to your regular practice at least three times a week: pigeon (or starfish) with Rooster Comb Hold (page 183), Spleen strengthen (page 184), and three-point Kidney (page 121). If you have cramps or breast tenderness, try belt flow (page 179). You can also do simple stretches to open up the stomach to help with cramps: lift your arms up overhead; hold on to your left wrist with your right hand, pulling your arms and waist over to the right (see page 137 in wood practice). Stand holding the back of a chair and stretch one foot back behind you until you feel a gentle stretch in your belly. (Adapted from *Energy Medicine for Women* by Donna Eden.)

9

Metal

The last turn on the wheel is autumn, the element metal. This is the end of the cycle before we move back into water and it all starts again. This is the time of harvest, of reaping what we've sown, but also a time of death, when the last leaves fall from the tree, leaving it bare and empty.

The challenge of metal is letting go. And for so many of us, this is the hardest lesson of all. Indeed, the Buddha said that the cause of all suffering is our attachment to impermanence—we become attached to the very things in life that change, such as people, situations, and even life itself. It is not the impermanence of life itself that causes suffering, but our attachment to it. When we see the world as it truly is—cycles upon cycles of passing time, where nothing lasts and change is the only constant—we are more able to find peace and contentment. Of course, this is the hardest lesson to master. To have deep, meaningful connections, we need to attach to people, places, things. It is this intensity of feeling that brings us such joy and satisfaction in life. And then, on the flip side, it is that very same intensity of feeling that leads to such incredible despair when we lose that to which we've been devoted. It is a paradox to which there is no answer.

I am not a Buddhist, and I have seen very few people, including the many I've known who practice Buddhism, who are not attached to the passages of this world. Instead, what I propose, is that we learn how to work with and transmute our emotions, our grief, and our pain. I really cannot see any other way for us to live fully and richly as humans and not be destroyed by our losses, but rather be inspired by what we've loved so much.

Transmuting grief and loss is not easy. It is perhaps the most difficult thing in the world: to understand, overcome, and live with trauma and grief. But it is also the single most important thing we must learn to do in order not to be annihilated by the exigencies of living.

The incredible shaman and teacher Martin Prechtel spoke of this so elo-quently in his powerful talk on grief and praise at a conference in Minneapolis. In his language, the word for grief and praise is one and the same. He says we must learn to grieve properly, that is, to fully abandon ourselves to the devasta-tion of our loss at the same time as exalting and praising the loss that we loved so much. This idea, of immersing ourselves in love for our loss, and letting our-selves feel that loss so deeply, is the key to transforming it into J. R. R. Tolkien's idea of punishments as gifts. The reason this is so difficult in our world, Prechtel says, is because we lack the community in which to do this. We lack the ability to completely lose ourselves in the moment of grieving and praising because we don't have the support of the tribe to both witness our journey and to make sure we don't drown in our process.[1]

One of the most powerful things you can do for transforming your own grief and loss is to have a witness. That might be a prayer group, a grieving support group, a family member, or a dear friend. The requisite need of this group is trust and a willingness of others to witness huge pain without trying to "fix" or change your emotional response.

The meridians that govern metal are Lung and Large Intestine. They are both organs of release, releasing toxins from opposite ends of our body. The lungs, in particular, hold grief, and it is no secret that in yoga, working with your lungs in the powerful pranayama practices is the key to the entire mind-body connection.

The Psychology of Metal

Metal people are organized, systematic, and straight shooters to the point that they can be dismissive or insensitive. But at the same time, they're the ones you want on your team when you need to get things figured out and done right. Their weakness can be that when the inevitable chaos of life intrudes, they're hamstrung. And they can be intolerable of others' emotionality. Metals need help lightening up, softening the exacting corners, and letting go.

Metals are analytical and when out of balance can be overly analytical. When in balance, metals can help us see the smooth surface below the emotionality of a situation. For us to let go of our trauma, we most often need to let go of the story. The emotions themselves, once the story is taken away, only last for a finite amount of time, time for the energy to run through the physiological expression of the story. Metals have the cool, Spock-like quality of being able to see clearly without the emotion. They know at some point, maybe far into the future, they're going to feel alright about this or that situation. Metals have the ability to get to this okay place sooner, and easier, often dispensing with the interim time of suffering. This is not denial of the situation. We have to be able to feel and process, harvest information, and let the emotion run through us. The trick is to let it run through and not get stuck in the story, which will keep running on an endless loop if we let it. When we have strong metal, we can see things rationally and can understand things without taking them personally. We can learn, move forward, and still stay connected to our life force.

The Physiology of Metal

The poses that help support and balance metal are backbends and twists. Twisting shows the physical body where the imbalances lie and helps bring the body into equilibrium while moving toxins, including emotional toxins. The metal backbends are softer and more supported than the ones in fire, which are about opening the heart to joy. Here, we are opening the heart to release pain so we can let joy back in. It is also an opening of the heart to loss, to heartache, to sadness. They both require opening. This is the challenge of metal. After grief, our natural tendency is to shut down. But doing that is in effect the end of our lives—and the trauma and grief we experienced are the last things we'll have. It takes courage to release the pain, which brings us to the next element, water. Metal prepares us to go back to the courage of living life, which we now know, with the wisdom of the end of the wheel, will be difficult and that more pain will come along. But the wisdom that we gain at the end of the wheel is that joy will also come and that grief and praise are two sides of the same coin. That is the balancing effect of the control cycle between metal and fire. Fire helps soften and shape metal. By bringing in the inspiration and joy of fire, we are led to the inspiration of metal. This is a different kind of inspiring. This is the inspiring of the breath—the in-and-out pulse of breath from the lungs that helps us temper and heal the soreness of our souls.

The sound to help release grief and balance the meridians associated with it is *sssss*.

The movement that helps us bridge the distance of metal to water is a bursting out. As with an intense emotional outbreak that soon subsides into gentle crying, we have a big expansion, which then contracts back into the tightly bound form of water. It's the big burst to return to the little burst. And the cycle starts again.

Metal Properties

Governs	Skin, hair
Season	Autumn
Meridians	Lung (yin), Large Intestine (yang)
Archetypes	The alchemist
Main Emotion	Challenging: Grief Balancing: Letting go, inspiration

The EMYoga Metal Practice

1 Wake Up

Start with a seated Wake Up. See page 78 for instructions and the online video.

2 Pranayama

Do sama vritti three to five minutes (see directions on page 69).

3 Massage Lung Neurolymphatic Reflex Points

In a seated, cross-legged position, deeply massage along the centerline of your sternum and one inch on either side of your sternum between your ribs. These are Lung neurolymphatic points, and releasing them will help you breathe deeper and oxygenate your lungs.

4 Deep Breath with Lengthened Exhale

Lengthen the exhale breath so it is longer than the inhale breath. Do ten breaths like this.

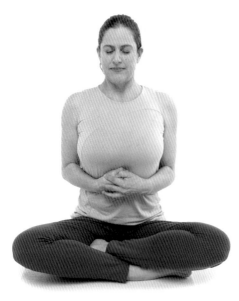

5 Free the Diaphragm

Make a fist with one hand and place it at the bottom of your rib cage in the center. Cup your other hand over it. Inhale and hold your breath, pressing your fist and your elbows into your body and your body into your arms. Exhale and release. Do this two more times. This builds lung capacity.

6 Hold on the Exhale

Kumbhaka Pranayama

Add a hold at the end of your exhale. Inhale slowly and deeply. Exhale slowly and deeply for a longer count than the inhale, then hold your breath out with your empty lungs for one or two counts. Repeat ten times.

7 Clear Metal Neurolymphatic Reflex Points on Thighs

Lie on your back and fold your knees into your chest. Make your hands into fists and deeply massage them into the "side seam" of your leg, on the outside and the inside. If you tend toward loose stools, massage from your knee to your hip. If you tend toward constipation, massage from your hip to your knee. Work as deeply as you can, even though this will be painful.

8 Leg in the Air Hamstring Stretch

Supta Padangusthasana

Lengthen your legs to the floor and
lift your right leg up into the air.
Place a strap around the sole of your
foot and hold the strap with both
hands. You can also hold your
big toe in a yogic toe lock if
you can easily reach it. Bring
your leg far enough up that you
feel a stretch in your hamstring. Try
to engage the quad, the opposing
muscle. Stay here for one minute.

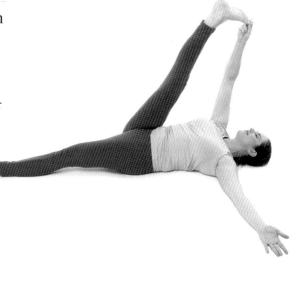

9 Leg Out to Side

Transfer the strap, or your foot, into
your right hand and open your leg
out to the right. You can lower
your leg as far down to the
floor as feels good. Press your
left hip bone down with your
left hand to make sure it doesn't
come up and misalign your body.
Hold one minute.

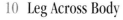

10 Leg Across Body

Bring your leg back up to center,
and switch the strap, or
your handhold, to your left
hand. Draw your leg across
your body down to the left side. Stay
up to one minute. Return to center
and repeat the sequence on the other
side. Then release down to the floor.

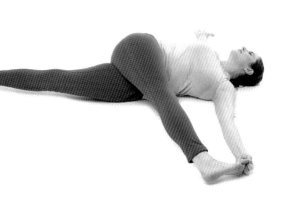

11 Slow Sit-Ups with Hook Up

Do slow sit-ups with no momentum. See page 92 for a detailed description. When you're complete, roll onto your belly and press to downward dog or child's pose to release. See the online video.

12 Alternating Arm and Leg Locust

Salabhasana

Lie on your belly. Bring your legs together and your arms to your low back with the back of your hands on your sacrum. Circle your hands around on your sacrum several times. Inhale and lift your left leg up while sweeping your right arm forward and up; lift your head, neck, and shoulders. Sweep your right arm back to the low back, release your leg down, and release your right cheek to the floor. Then switch sides. Lift your right leg up and sweep your left arm up until it is straight out in front of you. Head, neck, and shoulders also lift. Release down and release your left cheek to the floor. Do this three times each side. Then relax down and circle your hands around on your low back above your sacrum.

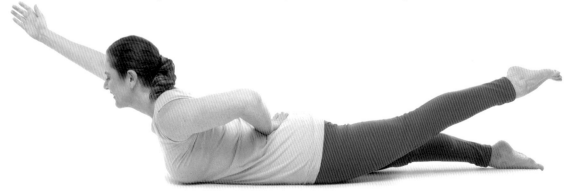

13 Full Locust with Heart Opener

Salabhasana

Still lying on your belly, lift both legs up, keeping them pressed together.
Lift both arms up lengthwise in front of you. Now bend your elbows
and bring your elbows back, hands in line with your shoulders creating a
"goalpost" with your arms. Let this movement "seat" your shoulder blades
deeper into your spine and open up the front of your heart. Hold three
to five breaths. Release.

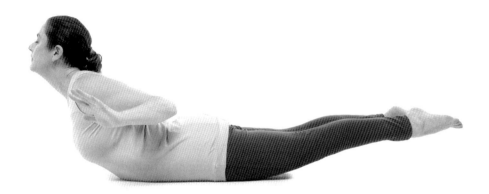

14 Cat-Cow

Come onto your hands and knees
and release your back with a few
cat-cows.

15 Downward Dog

Adho Mukha Svanasana

Press back into downward dog for
a few breaths. Then walk your feet
in and hang in a standing forward
bend for a breath, and slowly roll
up to stand.

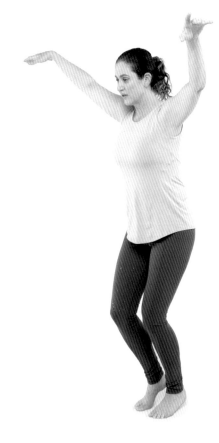

16 Heel Pounds: Shock Release

From standing, start to pound one heel and then the other onto the floor. You can lift your whole foot off the floor, or keep your toes on the floor. Keep pounding your heels harder and harder, and faster and faster. You can let your arms lift up overhead or keep them at your side. Let your whole body jiggle and wiggle. Pound your heels hard and make sound as loudly as feels good. Let this be a cathartic release. When you feel ready, begin to slow down, then come to stillness. Close your eyes and feel the continued shaking of your body. This is one of the ways animals "shake off" and release trauma.

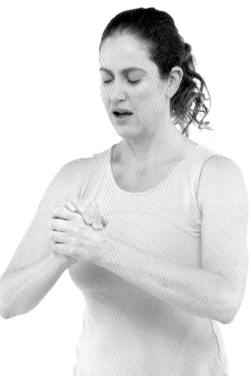

17 Hands Clench Jaw Shake

While standing, grasp your hands together in front of your body. Let your lower jaw separate from your upper jaw. Start to shake your gripped hands vigorously, forward and back, in front of your body. Let your jaw flap up and down. It can be very difficult to let go of the jaw, as this is the strongest muscle in the body. Start out slowly so the release happens. You might feel silly. But this helps release tension and stress from the entire head and jaw. See the online video.

18 Chair with Penetrating Flow

Utkatasana

See directions on page 85.

19 Belt Flow

See directions on page 179.

20 Forward Wide-Leg Bend with Twist

Prasarita Padottanasana

From standing, separate your feet about three feet apart and turn them parallel. Inhale, with your hands on your hips, and lift your heart up. Exhale and release your body halfway forward so your spine is parallel with the floor. Take one breath and release your body all the way forward. If you can reach your feet easily, place the first two fingers from each hand on the toenail bed of each big toe. Take five to ten breaths. You can have a slight bend in the back of your knee. Then gently twist each side by placing your right hand in the center and lifting your left arm to the sky. Hold three to five breaths and switch, placing your left hand in the center and your right hand up in the air. Take three to five breaths. Rest in the center, and then slowly come up, tracing Spleen.

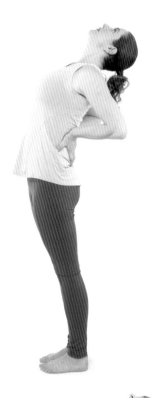

21 Supported Standing Backbend

Stand in tadasana with your body balanced, left to right and front to back. Lift your sternum, opening your heart, and lift your head to the sky. Feel the muscles in your back, below your shoulder blades, supporting the pose. Now bring your hands to your low back, and open and lift your heart a bit more with the increased support your arms offer. Make sure you feel no strain. If your neck is straining, don't drop your head so far back. Hold here for several breaths, making sure your breath is smooth and easy and not straining at all. Come back to tadasana.

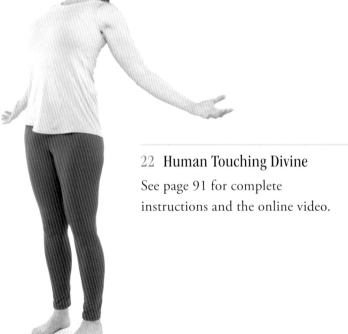

22 Human Touching Divine

See page 91 for complete instructions and the online video.

23   Blowing Out the Candle

Slowly lower down to a squat (you won't need your padding here, as you'll be here only briefly). Wrap one arm around your knees, and let the other come in front of you for balance. Inhale, looking down. Exhale, look up, and audibly exhale with the sound *whoooo*. Do that two more times. Then release onto hands and knees.

24   Cat-Cow

Release your spine by alternating arching and sinking your spine as you deeply breathe.

25   All Fours to Arm-Leg Opposite Extension

From all fours, extend your left leg along the floor, first with your toes tucked under, stretching the back of your leg. Then lift your leg, keeping it parallel to the floor, in line with your body. Extend your right arm out in front of you, also parallel to the floor. Hold for three to five breaths. Switch sides.

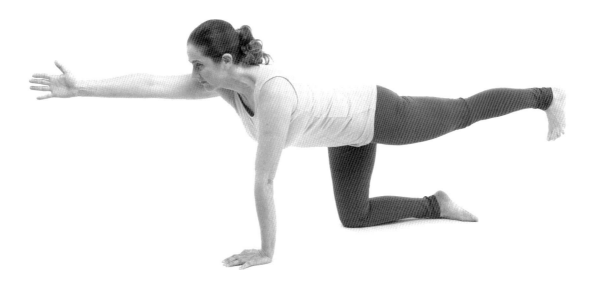

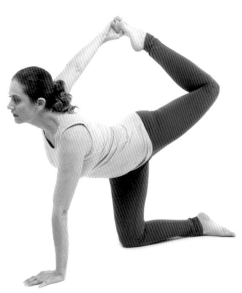

26 Loop and Hold Opposite Leg

Now bend your left knee and reach around behind you with your right arm to hold your left ankle. Press your foot away from your body, increasing the opening in your heart. If you can, press your thumb or fingers into Kidney 1 as you hold your foot. Hold three to five breaths. Release, and repeat on the other side.

27 Downward Dog to Long Hold Plank to Side Hold Plank

Adho Mukha Svanasana to Vasisthasana

Come into downward dog. Take three breaths. Come forward to plank pose. Hold here five to ten breaths. Release to side plank on the right side, balancing on your right hand and the outside of your right foot. Lift your left arm up, and avoid sagging in your hips. Hold five to ten breaths. Repeat on the other side. Come back to downward dog.

28 Bean with Head Heal

Release your body in child's pose for several breaths. Place your hands one on top of the other and rest your head in your hands. Now slowly come forward onto your elbows and bring your face to rest in your hands, with the heels of your hands on your cheekbones and your palms over your eye sockets. Stay here one minute.

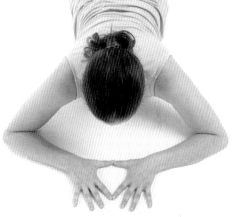

29 Downward-Facing Triple Diamond

This pose is for releasing grief and sadness. Lie on your stomach with your knees out to the sides and the soles of your feet touching. Bring your thumbs and index fingers to touch in front of you, and rest the bridge of your nose on your thumbs. You may need to stack your thumbs to avoid squishing your nose. Elbows are out to the sides. Remain here as long as feels good. To come out of the pose, lengthen your arms and legs and roll them in their sockets, then roll over onto your back and hug your knees into your chest.

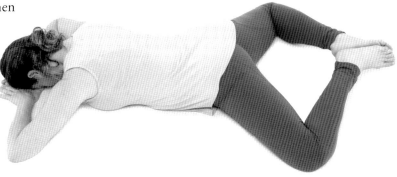

30 Moving Bridge with Metal Neurolymphatic Clear

Dwi Pada Pitham

Follow instructions for moving bridge on page 94. Deeply massage the Lung points following the centerline of your sternum and the line one inch on either side of the centerline and the Large Intestine points along the outer thighs. Exhale with a *sssss*.

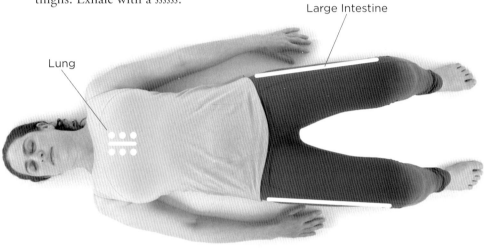

Large Intestine

Lung

31 Wheel

Urdhva Dhanurasana

If you practice wheel, come up into it now. If you don't practice wheel, you can come back up into bridge, this time rolling your shoulders under your back to open your upper back more. Stay in either pose three to five breaths. Come down to rest for three breaths. And come up one more time.

32 Supported Shoulder Stand or Legs Up the Wall with Electrics

Sarvangasana or Viparita Karani

See detailed instructions on page 96.
Rest here for two to ten minutes.

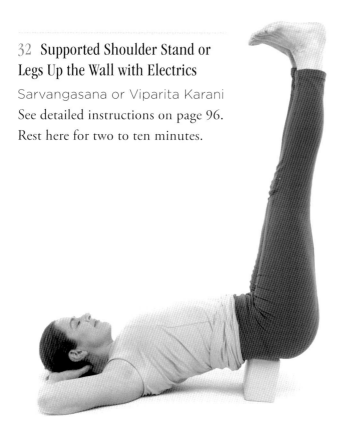

33 Plow

Halasana

Fold a blanket and lie on your back so your shoulders are on the blanket, head off. Lift your legs in the air. Bring them as far overhead as is comfortable. Massage your calves here from the backs of your knees to your Achilles tendons, then rest your hands on the backs of the knees. Stay several breaths, then slowly lower down and hug your knees to your chest.

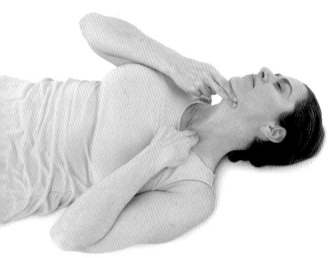

34 Fish with Chakra Clear

Matsyasana

See full instructions on page 97 and the online video. *Note:* If you're used to releasing your hands from the floor in fish, you can clear the chakra channels while up in the full pose. *If any of those channels are sore or calling for your attention, you'll use that one chakra in the next pose.*

35 Circle Calling Chakra

You'll work with the chakra that called your attention most in the prior pose. Locate the corresponding chakra from the throat channel and bring one hand over that chakra (see page 99 for chakra locations). You can be touching your body, or slightly off your body. Or you can start with your hand far off your body and slowly lower it toward your body until you feel a slight "resistance" energetically. Begin to make circles over the chakra in a counterclockwise direction. If your hand gets tired, you can switch hands. You might feel moved to shake off the energy every so often. You might feel warmth, heat, tingling, or other sensations. You might also get images or information. Continue circling two to three minutes. Then shake off your hand and start to circle in the other direction. Continue circling for two to three minutes clockwise, and then relax your arm to the side.

Note: If you are working on the crown chakra, and you are a man, you'll start the circling in a clockwise direction, and then conclude in a counterclockwise direction. All other chakras start counterclockwise and end clockwise.

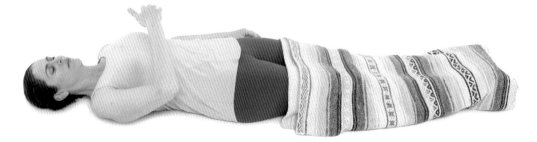

36 Chakra Link

Choose another chakra whose information or essence could help support the chakra you've been working with. (See basic chakra info on page 101.) For example, if you've been working with the root chakra (your home, tribe, grounding), perhaps you'll bring in the energy of the heart chakra, infusing the root with love, acceptance, and joy.

Place one hand over the original chakra you were working with, and place your other hand over the chakra you chose to connect. Hold here for two to three minutes. Support your arms with props so you can relax here. You may feel warmth or buzzing.

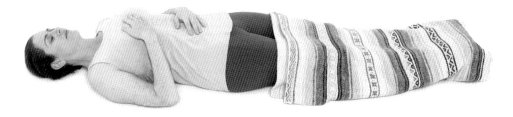

37 Savasana Prep with Metal Neurovascular Reflex Points Hold

Before you release into final savasana, place one hand across your forehead and the other on the top of your head. Use props so you can relax here. Hold here one to three minutes, and then release into full savasana.

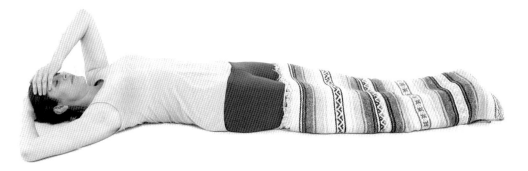

38 Savasana

Relax completely for five to fifteen minutes.

39 Pranayama: Sama Vritti

In a comfortable cross-legged seat, allow your breath to deepen and equalize again into a sama vritti pattern (see page 128). Now increase the length of your exhale breath. Add the sound *sssss* to your breath. Continue for one to three minutes. Release the breathing pattern and let your breath return to normal.

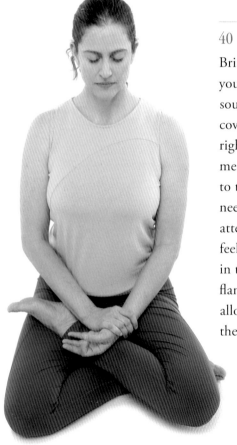

40 Meditation

Bring your left hand loosely into your lap. Hold the Lung and Heart source points on your left hand by covering your inner wrist with your right hand as you do the following meditation. Bring your awareness to the primary chakra that was in need of attention above. Rest your attention there. Allow yourself to feel a warmth or pulsing sensation in that chakra. Visualize a golden flame at the chakra center. Stay here, allowing your attention to remain on the chakra for five to fifteen minutes.

PART 3

Spirit

Energy Medicine Yoga Off the Mat

∞

Athletic, artistic, and intellectual performance is
enhanced when all of the body's communication
channels are open and balanced . . . to facilitate the
progress of individuals in their personal evolution . . .
in the achievement of their personal goals or "destiny."

JAMES L. OSCHMAN
Energy Medicine

10

Ayurveda and Diet

EMYoga reaches into every area of life and shows us that there is no *one* way to live, to practice yoga, to thrive, or to heal the body. The prescription for healing is a composite. Working with issues on the physical level (asanas, diet, body care), mental level (emotions, feelings, thoughts), and spiritual level (meditation, journaling, gratitude) helps find the spark that will change a disease pattern back into a healthy pattern. In this chapter, I share some Ayurvedic tools and my dietary suggestions to support healing and optimal energy.

Top Three Ayurvedic Tools
That Will Change Your Life Right Now

Following are my favorite three tools from Ayurveda, the medicinal arm of yoga, which will have a huge positive and immediate effect on your health. They are simple and have an enormous payback in terms of calming and healing the nervous system and all the energy systems of the body.

1. NASYA

Nasya is the practice of oiling the nasal cavity. Your nose is the gateway not only to your entire respiratory track, ending in the delicate tissue of your lungs, but it is also a direct pathway to your brain. The nerves in your nose connect directly to the brain and are the only nerves in the body that can regenerate. This direct connection to the brain is why the sense of smell is the most powerfully linked to both memory and emotion. When you inhale something, it goes to the olfactory bulb and then directly to the limbic system, which is where memory and moods are processed. You also have more receptors for smell than for any other sense.[1]

The nostrils are just tiny openings to a larger system composed of thin bony plates called turbinates. Located deep inside the navel cavity, turbinates are lined with millions of tiny hairs called cilia, which defend the body against irritants and contagions in the air. As we breathe in, the air is circulated through these turbinates where it is warmed and cleaned before it descends into our lungs. The turbinates are our main interface with the world around us, including all the toxins, illnesses, bacteria, dryness, and humidity—in other words, our environment. They also help deepen our breath, allowing a fully oxygenated belly breath instead of the stress-inducing chest breathing that so many people do.

When you do the nasya technique, you are helping to keep the turbinates healthy, which has a variety of beneficial effects on the head and neck. Primarily, nasya is a guard against pathogens entering the body. By effectively coating the cilia in a desired oil, you build a healthy barrier against unwanted toxins. This adds a deep flexibility to your interface with the world, building resilience.

Nasya helps clear and lubricate the sinus passageways, relieving acute and chronic sinus problems, such as allergies, mucous congestion, dry nasal passages, and snoring. Nasya also helps relieve headaches, migraines, stiff neck, fatigue, insomnia, and stress-related problems.[2]

This is one of the easiest, quickest, and most powerful tools you can add to your daily routine, and it is indeed a life changer.

Because of the power of the sense of smell and the brain connection, you can also choose particular scents to achieve particular outcomes. You can use organic sesame oil, but do not use straight, undiluted, essential oils in the nose, as they are far too strong. Purchase an oil specifically created for nasya. There are resources in the back of the book for finding them.

LEARN TO DO NASYA

This technique feels amazing. It is not harsh like using a neti pot. It is quite comfortable and enjoyable. So don't be afraid. Lie on your back with a pillow or some support under your neck and shoulders so your nostrils are pointing up. Hold the oil dropper over your nostrils. You can place the tip of the dropper on the inside of the nostril to help you get your bearings before dropping the oil in. You can also ask for help from a friend to figure it out the first time. It may take some practice, but once you get the hang of it, it's really quite simple. Exhale completely and then place one to three drops in each nostril. You can do one side at a time, or both together. After you've dropped the oil in, sniff up strongly several times, pinching and releasing the nostrils to bring the oil deep into the nasal cavities, which extend all the way up above your eyes, as well as deep on both sides of your nose. You can help bring the oils up by massaging along the sides of the nose, between and above the eyebrows, and under the eyes. Lie on your back for a minute or two before getting up. If you get up too soon, you might get postnasal drip. If that happens, stay longer on your back next time. See the online video.

IS YOUR CELL PHONE TOXIC?

In *Spontaneous Healing*, Andrew Weil writes: "Electromagnetic pollution may be the most significant form of pollution human activity has produced in this century, all the more dangerous because it is invisible and insensible."[3]

Recent findings from studies by the National Toxicology Program state that cell phone radiation increases cancer rates in rats and mice.[4]

Here is what happens to your cells when they are assaulted by EMF waves, as explained to me by biophysical practitioner and educator Brett Tallman:

The radio signals that are coming from wireless devices are microwaves, which are long waves, but on the back of those waves are piggybacked tiny short waves that happen to be the same size as your cells, and they're coming at you in a rapid staccato-like fashion. Because they're the same size as your cells, your cells see them as a threat. The cellular body then constricts like a sea anemone might if you touch it; it stays constricted, hardens up, and shuts down for up to several hours after exposure. When that happens, cell respiration stops, which means the cell stops letting nutrients in and toxins out. Cell-to-cell communication starts to break down as the signaling mechanisms, such as chemicals and light waves, are no longer transmitted or received. This shutting down of the cell results in DNA damage due to toxin buildup within the cell. The cell wants to stay alive. Even if it can't detox or respire, it still wants to live. If it doesn't oxygenate for a long time, it turns into a cancer cell. The signaling from the wireless devices is like a master toxin. If you have a preexisting weakness or toxic buildup in your body, it'll make it worse.[5]

There are many ways to mitigate the onslaught of cell towers and Wi-Fi. Many companies make devices that interrupt and scramble these "coherent" frequencies to allow our bodies to identify and protect against them. You can find resources for these at the back of the book. This is the simplest and most important first step to protect yourself. If you can hardwire the computers in your home, and/or turn off the Wi-Fi at night, you can also help protect yourself. There are several groups that are actively trying to get Wi-Fi out of schools, especially for young children, who are at the greatest risk.

2. SELF-ABHYANGA

The newest cutting-edge science on health and disease is research into the gut-brain axis. Our gut is considered the second brain. The gut creates more neurotransmitters than the brain, including 95 percent of our serotonin, the neurotransmitter that helps us sleep and regulates our moods. There is now scientific proof that our "gut reaction" is in fact a real thing.[6]

The "atmosphere" of the gut is now considered another organ. It is called the microbiome. And the science being done around it is perhaps the most bizarre and interesting in terms of disease control and reversal.

The microbiome is made up of the microbes that symbiotically live with the human. There are more microbial cells than any other kind of cell in the body, so cell for cell we're all just big bugs. Lucky for us, the microbial cells are much smaller and encompass only 1 to 3 percent of our body weight. But the power of these tiny cells cannot be overstated.

Our gut, along with the intestinal linings that includes our esophagus and our mouth, is made of the same skin as the skin on the outside of our body. It just continues on into the inside, down our throat, into our belly. These microbial beings in our guts are also all over the outside of our bodies, on our skin. The healthier these microbes are, the healthier we are. And although the research on this fascinating "new organ" is being done today, five thousand years ago Ayurvedic doctors knew how important this was.

The Ayurvedic sages came up with a technique that is one of my top three. It is called abhyanga, or self-massage using warm body oil. In order to soothe and feed your billions of microbes, you oil your skin. Among its many other benefits beyond that, abhyanga:

- releases the powerful neurotransmitter oxytocin, which is the love hormone, making you feel happier, more loving, and more compassionate—toward yourself as well as others

- helps facilitate the direction of energy flowing in your body (when using EMYoga meridian pathways)

- helps keep your skin young and supple

- helps your joints with increased blood circulation

- boosts the immune system

- helps resolve emotional issues through contact with the skin, which connects directly to the brain's limbic system

Use only organic oil. Traditionally sesame oil is used, but you can use coconut oil, almond oil, avocado oil, or anything you're drawn to, including scented oils. The only parameter is that the oils are organic because your body is literally "eating" the oil.

SELF-ABHYANGA THE EMYOGA WAY

Heat some oil by placing the bottle in warm water. Stand in a warm bathroom on a towel or mat. Pour some oil in your hands, and starting at the outside edges of your big toes, smooth up the inside of your legs to your groins, and then smooth around and down the outsides of your legs. You'll do this as many times as feels good, stopping at your knees either on the way up or the way down, and making circles around the joints. You can also do circles around the ankle bones.

Spend a few extra moments massaging between the bones of your toes and in between your toes to "clear the gates" and move excess meridian energy from your body. Also, do several swipes from your buttocks down the backs of your legs. Stop at the backs of your knees (the popliteal crease) and massage deeply there before continuing down.

Take one hand with oil and massage from the backs of your fingertips up to your shoulders, then swipe around to your armpit and smooth down the inside of your arm and off your palm. Do this several times, stopping at your elbows and shoulders, making circles around the joints. Massage your hands, and clear the gates on your hands as well as pulling off the end of each fingertip.

Smooth oil on your belly and circle first in a clockwise direction, then counterclockwise. Be sure to do this lovingly, as the belly is often a place that is disliked, especially for women. Take this opportunity to literally tell your body you're giving it a treat, both the skin and the gut!

Smooth oil around both breasts, and circle in both clockwise and counterclockwise directions. It is also nice to do a large figure eight around both breasts. Use this opportunity to do a self-exam on your breasts. The more you know the landscape of your breasts, the more you are able to find any changes that might require further attention. When you are done oiling and checking your breasts, squeeze them. Squeezing the breasts helps realign cancerous cells into a normal cell structure.[7]

Squeeze the top of one shoulder and swipe down to the opposite hip on the front of your body. Do this on both sides several times.

With oil, make circles in both directions on each butt cheek. Continue making circles and figure eights on your low back for as far up as you can reach.

Smooth oil on your neck, and smooth the skin outward in all directions as well as up and down the "chakra channels" of your throat.

Gently run your fingertips over your face, smoothing upward. Make figure eights around your eye sockets. Smooth your fingers on either side of your jawbone.

Rub some oil on your fingertips and massage your fingers deep into your scalp, paying close attention to any sore areas. Massage these sore areas even more. You can wash your hair when you get in the bath, and the oil is quite good for your roots too.

After you've covered your whole body with oil, you can then go into the shower or bath, carefully, as you might be slippery! The warm water will drive the oil deeper into your skin. Do not wash the oil off. You can use soap on your genitals, anus, and armpits, but allow the oil to remain on your skin. Dry off by patting your body with a towel.

Although it is preferable to do this before you bathe, you can also do this entire sequence after your shower or bath. You might want to pat off the oil then, before you dress.

3. THREE MEALS A DAY, NO SNACKS

Diet is a central tenet of Ayurvedic healing. Not only what you eat, but when and how. This simple Ayurvedic philosophy helps weight loss, digestive issues, depression, balances blood sugar, and reduces cravings. It also helps people come into their natural best weight. It is remarkably easy, yet at the same time, in this day and age of constant eating, it can be very challenging to practice.

TRY EATING THE AYURVEDIC WAY

Three meals a day. No snacks.

That's it. Three meals a day. No snacks.

Sounds pretty easy, right?

My first dismissal of this seemingly easy philosophy was because I am a snacker. I ate every few hours, or even more. I subscribed to the snack industry's adamant nutritional council that you should eat ten small meals a day. I work hard outside, skiing, hiking, whatever-ing, and I need to constantly fuel my body. I have low blood sugar; I can't go more than two hours without eating. On and on went my reasons why I couldn't possibly try this out. But I was struggling with stomachaches again, something that had plagued me during my years of nonstop international travel—and I was getting desperate.

It was Thanksgiving. As we were clearing the meal, I started to pick some skin off the turkey, and my best friend and Ayurvedic practitioner, Elaine Doll, gently pointed out the habit I wasn't even aware of. Then she explained the reasoning.

When you finish eating a meal (indeed, while you're still eating), your body is putting together the enzymes it will use to digest it. It takes all the food, now chewed up into a ball of mush, and starts the difficult process of digesting it and absorbing its nutrients. This takes an enormous amount of energy, which is why we so often get tired after eating. Your body is digesting away, and two hours later or twenty minutes later, you toss down some cookies, an apple, or a smoothie. Now your body has to turn away from the work it was doing to digest your last meal and start the work of digesting this new food, leaving the prior meal mid-digestion, or, as they say in the medical lingo, putrefying. If you continue to do that, hour after hour, your body never fully digests everything, and it is constantly working. Your body never has a chance to do all the other things it needs to do because it is working on digesting.

The body is built to burn stored fat for its energy. If you are constantly feeding it new sugars, it will burn those for energy, and it loses its ability to burn fat, which is the slow-burning, constant form of energy the body craves. Instead, it is using the fresh stuff you keep throwing at it. This is what causes energy crashes, cravings, depression, and all sorts of imbalances. Exhaustion and fatigue happen on a physical level when the body is always digesting. You are taking the body out of its natural working ability and forcing it to behave the way Nabisco wants it to behave.

When you first go to three meals a day, no snacks, you may feel strange. You may feel hungry in between meals. If so, eat a bigger meal next time to give your body the fuel to make it to your next meal. You may feel anxious or moody. You can eat four meals a day initially if blood sugar is really challenged, so long as there are at least three hours in between, then gradually move to three meals only. Notice how much food and eating brings you back to your childhood eating patterns. What was mealtime like at your house? What was snack time like? How did you cope with challenges? Did you eat?

I started this program the day after Thanksgiving. At first it was difficult. I noticed my impulse to reach for something to eat each time I walked past the kitchen, whether or not I was hungry. I noticed extreme anxiety at meals. That first week I ate huge meals to assure myself I wouldn't get hungry in between. But very soon that leveled off, and I came to know the balance of how much food my body wanted. I started to feel incredibly empowered at my ability to resist the constant munching I saw around me. It was the holidays, and there were treats everywhere. But I was simply unmoved by even the gooiest, stickiest, yummiest treat. On the annual cookie stroll downtown, I brought a lunch bag and took cookies from every shop. I ate them all for breakfast the next morning! With a big glass of raw milk. (Every once in a while, indulging in sugar is okay in my book!)

Another powerful component is giving yourself the love and care of preparing a meal and then sitting down to eat and enjoy it. In our age of takeout and car eating, constant snacking, and life on the go, this is a reclaiming of what was once communal and nurturing, indeed a sacred time.

However, the biggest thing of all—the thing that has kept me on this "diet" for almost two years, and will keep me on it for life—is that it works. From day one, I completely stopped having stomachaches. And I haven't had another one since, not even on a cookies-for-breakfast morning!

A Healthy EMYoga Diet

Let food be thy medicine and medicine be thy food.

HIPPOCRATES

At this particular point in time in our culture, the word *diet* usually means restricting our caloric intake with the aim of losing weight. It also often means a restriction of certain foods, with the aim generally being the same, to lose weight. It has only recently broadened out in the past several years with various eating plans to address other health issues, including blood pressure, heart health, mood, diabetes, allergies, and more.

But what is generally not talked about in the diet magazines and books is how food affects us both physically and mentally. How do you feel in your body when you eat this or that? How do you feel while it digests and moves through your body, and when it is eliminated? Almost no one talks about the energetics of food. Food that is fresh, alive, and health giving has a vibration that is easier for the body to assimilate. Food that is prepackaged and processed is more difficult for the body to digest. Processed food is also high in sugars, unhealthy fats, and is generally not "alive." In Ayurveda, foods that have a fatigue-inducing, detrimental effect are considered *tamasic*.

Feeling is a primary sensor of a healthy diet. It doesn't matter what you look like, it matters how you feel. Are you flexible and strong? Do you have resiliency? Can you get sick and then get well? Are you strong enough to accomplish the task at hand? How do you feel? The food you eat is what makes you. It literally becomes you. But when we talk about diet, we so often just mean how much we eat or don't eat.

Food is nurturing and satisfies our basic urges. It is the connective tissue of our families. It ties us back to our ancestors. It is also a mainstay of social interactions. But this is not always a positive thing. And many of us struggle with eating as a result of how we ate growing up.

When we eat for feeling instead of eating for taste, or comfort, or to be part of our tribe, we are on the path of balance. It isn't easy. Food is a powerful substance, as we know, especially if we've fallen into the bucket of ice cream after a breakup or the slabs of pizza out with friends. I certainly don't mean to say we shouldn't find pleasure in food. Eating can be one of the most pleasurable experiences we have. But when we only feel the pleasure in our mouths and not in our entire being, we can succumb to the imbalance of the addict.

There is a lot of confusion in the diet and nutrition world. Facts change as new studies come out, negating years of accepted practice in an instant. For years there was a huge push on nonfat foods, and no one could figure out why everyone was getting fatter and fatter. Then we learned that fat isn't bad for us, but there are different kinds of fat. And cholesterol isn't bad for us, but there are different kinds of cholesterol. Some aspects of soy, in certain forms, may protect against cancer, while others may cause cancer. The jury is still out. There is a general consensus that sugar is bad across the board. But there is no consensus about alcohol, caffeine, chocolate, dairy, animal protein, or green tea.

Compounding this problem is that a huge percentage of this "bad" information comes from certified nutritionists, MDs, PhDs, and people credentialed in all sorts of ways, giving them the sheen of authority. So people follow their advice. Then debunking that advice and reversing years of bad habits authoritatively given is extremely challenging. If we can't trust the "experts," who can we trust?

My answer: trust your energy! This is when energy testing becomes an invaluable tool (see page 30), and by doing your own research on yourself, you find the diet that works for you, not the diet that the experts say is today's best fix.

If you've read the top three Ayurvedic tools that will change your life, you already know my feelings about how and when to eat: three meals a day, no snacks.

There is a lot of wisdom (five thousand years!) in the Ayurvedic eating styles. There are many wonderful and easy books that share this wisdom. Among my favorites are Dr. John Douillard's *Body, Mind & Sport* and Deepak Chopra's *Perfect Health*. One of the simplest pieces of that wisdom you can follow without reading another diet book is this: eat seasonally. The seasons bring forth the foods we need when we need them. Spring shoots help cleanse the body from the heaviness of winter. Summer berries give us major antioxidants. Fall roots help us nourish and ground as we go into the long winter. It goes on . . . the wisdom of the seasons is once again in play for us.

Another Ayurvedic tool is to eat until you are three-quarters full. If you eat your meal with attention, you will notice a small burp. It might not be audible. It might just be a little air bubble coming up in between bites. This is the signal that your body has enough food. It is amazing; the little bubble is there every single meal you eat. Pay attention next time and see for yourself, and use that opportunity to stop eating.

This brings us to what to actually eat.

I don't like to spend hours preparing food or hours eating food. I like to nourish my body. I want to eat as healthily as I can and also enjoy what I eat. After studying diet and nutrition for years, using myself as a guinea pig, I've discovered a diet that works for me. This is what I'm going to share with you because all of my students ask me this question. This is not scientific. This is not double-blind studied and triple-fact-checked, but it is time-honored and sustainable. This is what my ancestors did and what I now do, and I'm sharing it with you.

Please note, if you have particular needs (diabetes, allergies, extreme body dysmorphia), I would suggest you work with a certified nutritionist, and perhaps even an Ayurvedic one, a practitioner who is flexible and up on the most recent studies and is not consumed with dogma. That is the biggest limitation to finding a system that truly works for you, your own dogma, or someone else's. As in every other section of this book, I urge you to question your assumptions, do your research, and come to your own conclusions.

Most of the foods I recommend are also recommended by some of the leading functional medical doctors of today, people such as Josh Axe and Andrew Weil, along with some guiding principles from Weston A. Price (a dentist best known for his research on nutrition), Sally Fallon (nutritional cookbook author), and the late, great Aajonus Vonderplanitz (a nutritionist and food rights activist).

This is my basic overview of a healing, nourishing, diet. The overarching principle through all of this is the use of organic foods, supplements, drinks, and herbs. For me, this is nonnegotiable. It is expensive, and it is where I spend the bulk of my money. But this is one area where I can exercise choice to limit my toxic intake significantly, as well as affect the supply chain, limiting toxic exposure to farmers, field workers, and packers. With that, I'll share with you the foods that work for me and my students.

FAT!

I was a victim of the nonfat fad in my early twenties. This, in my opinion, was the biggest deficit in my food plan, and led to overeating, weight gain, depression, and a general sense that I would never, ever, ever be calm and joyful around food but rather would be destined to struggle with my weight, struggle with my relationship with food, and feel out of control at any food-related event.

That all ended, instantaneously, when I discovered the secret that my great-grandmother, who lived to 101, knew all along. She was a dairy maid in Lithuania before she emigrated to the United States in 1910, and I have a huge debt of gratitude to her. This wisdom was passed on through the aether, to her granddaughter, my mother. Though a child of the 1950s, she became a countercultural rebel in the 1960s and 1970s, and her involvement with the New Age movement helped her create a food culture in my childhood household that I can only describe as "hippy." I hated it then: lentil burgers (we called them boogie burgers), vats of raw honey, vats of peanut butter, a buying co-op in our garage once a week, and, God bless her, raw milk.

It might have taken a couple decades for me to come back to what I learned as a child, but the beauty of ancestral wisdom is that it exists in our fields. The fact that I was weaned on raw milk—in my opinion the healthiest raw fat there is—is one of the reasons I have such a healthy constitution today.

Raw food pioneer and leading nutritionist Aajonus Vonderplanitz taught that "because fat cleanses, fuels, lubricates, and protects the body, it is needed more than any other single nutrient. . . . Fat is also a necessary catalyst for utilizing minerals and protein. . . . The body can, to some extent, turn sugars, starches, and proteins into fats, but not nearly enough, and it is a long and exhausting process on the body. When fats are eaten raw, they can and will clean, fuel, lubricate, and protect the body properly."[8]

Raw fats include unsalted raw butter, fertile eggs, raw cream and milk, unsalted raw cheese, the fat in and on all meats, fresh coconut, avocados, and olive oil (and other cold-pressed oils). Nuts and seeds are also raw fats but can be difficult to digest and should be soaked and sprouted first and eaten in moderation.

My personal preference for raw fat is predominantly dairy. I try to find raw, organic dairy wherever I live or travel. This is difficult at times due to government interference on the right to choose what we eat, but it can be done. You can go to RealMilk.com to find a list of offerings. Even in states where it is illegal, you can source raw dairy in many different ways. Cow shares and herd shares are two ways, and often there are people willing to sell to you if you find them at farmers markets or your local natural food store. Once, when I was living in Whitehorse, in the Yukon Territory of Canada, which has prohibitive raw dairy laws, I worked a trade with a blind goat farmer. I helped mend fences, took the herd on walks, and cleaned the dairy room, in exchange for my half gallon of fresh raw goat milk. It was more dear to me than gold!

Vonderplanitz explains the benefits of raw dairy this way: "The fat in raw cream and full-fat raw milk soothes and lubricates nerves and muscles, including the heart, gently cleanses and lubricates the liver, restores moisture to the thyroid, and heals intestinal lesions from dryness. The fat in unsalted raw butter strengthens organs and glands, heals eyes, cleanses arteries and [the] vascular system of plaque from hardened cooked fats, and lubricates bones, cartilage and teeth. It is utilized for all body-fat needs: cleansing, lubricating, fueling, protecting, rejuvenating, and reproducing cells."[9]

If you do not eat dairy, eat lots of avocados, olive oil (not cooked, but on salads, etc.), coconuts and coconut oil, and some seeds and nuts. For most people in North America, eating raw meat is often thought of as highly distasteful, and you're considered untrustworthy if you eat it. But call it another name and then you're fine. Sushi, which was once considered gross (Raw fish? Blech!), is now found in every strip mall in America and fish oil (fish fat) is all the rage as well. Steak tartar (raw hamburger), carpaccio (raw steak), and ceviche (raw fermented fish or meat) have always been in vogue in upscale restaurants and are eaten all over Europe. Organ meats (think pâté) are full of nutrients that benefit your body too. If you are not turned off by these foods, add them to your diet.

There are many teachers and disciplines that require or advise a vegetarian diet, using the yogic tenet of *ahimsa*, or nonviolence, to advocate this. My reading of ahimsa comes from yoga master T. K. V. Desikachar, who writes in *The Heart of Yoga*, "We must always behave with consideration and attention to others."[10] In my opinion, eating meat, cheese, or eggs that are from humanely raised and humanely slaughtered animals falls into that category.

RAW HONEY

This is the healthiest sweetener on the planet. It does not spike your blood sugar the way other sugars do (including maple syrup . . . sorry).

Medical Medium Anthony William writes this about honey:

> The sugar in honey is nothing like processed sugar—don't confuse it with table sugar or high-fructose corn syrup. Rather, because bees collect from plant species far and wide, the fructose

and glucose in honey are saturated with more than 200,000 undiscovered phytochemical compounds and agents, including pathogen-killers, phytochemicals that protect you from radiation damage, and anti-cancerous phytochemicals. When drawn into cancerous tumors and cysts, this last class of phytochemicals shut down the cancerous growth process—meaning that raw honey can stop cancer in its tracks. Honey's highly absorbable sugar and B12 coenzymes make it one of the most powerful brain foods of our time. Plus, raw honey repairs DNA and is extremely high in minerals such as calcium, potassium, zinc, selenium, phosphorus, chromium, molybdenum, and manganese.[11]

It has many other healing benefits as well. It is antimicrobial and antibacterial; it helps heal wounds and soothe the intestinal track. It is helpful for allergies, particularly if it is harvested locally. It includes many enzymes, which help digestion. It is the best alternative to other sugars, helping people transition away from them, while still enjoying sweetness.

SAUERKRAUT AND OTHER FERMENTED FOODS

These are among the best foods for helping heal and strengthen the microbiome (the culture of organisms that live and work both inside you and on your skin). They are some of the only foods that can actually change the microbiome. They contain live enzymes that help the body digest food and are some of the most life-giving beneficial foods you can eat.

Fermented foods other than sauerkraut include kimchee, kefir, yogurt (make sure you buy plain kefir or plain yogurt, as many varieties have incredibly high levels of added sugar).

The alternative food bible *Nourishing Traditions* says this about fermented foods:

Professor Zabel observed that sick people always lack digestive juices, not only during the acute phase of their illness but also for a longtime afterwards. In addition, he never saw a cancer victim that had a healthy intestinal flora. . . . Thus, the different lacto-fermented foods are a valuable aid to the cancer patient. They are rich in vitamins and minerals and contain as well enzymes that cancer patients lack. Of particular value are lacto-fermented beets, which have a very favorable effect on disturbed cellular function. Many scientific studies have demonstrated that beets have a regenerating effect on the body.[12]

SOURDOUGH

This is a subset of fermented foods because it is itself fermented. Sourdough (made the traditional way and allowed to sour for an extended period of time) is generally tolerated by those who complain of gluten intolerance because its fermentation process aids digestion.

TONICS

There are many delicious and health-giving tonics out there. I've experimented primarily with kombucha (made with a fermented "mother," or culture, called a SCOBY) and Kevita (made with the same "grains" used to make kefir, a fermented dairy drink). But my go-to, easiest-to-make and favorite drink is called switchel. You can make it easily by mixing raw honey, raw apple cider vinegar, and good clean well or spring water. Apple cider vinegar has more healing benefits than is possible to describe here. It helps with digestion, elimination, weight control, oxygenating the body, headaches, healing skin internally and externally . . . the list goes on. This is a power drink and is wonderful to have at hand.

BONE BROTH

This simple-to-make staple helps the body access collagen, vitamins, and important minerals that help the connective tissue, skin, bowels, bones, and brain. It also helps soothe and heal the digestive system. It is becoming more frequently available to purchase ready-made.

PASTURED, FERTILIZED RAW EGGS

I tend to eat my eggs raw, disguised in a raw milk smoothie. They are one of the easiest foods to digest and are a complete protein. If you are quite ill and cannot tolerate eating much, eggs can help you get back into health and strength. Some people, however, may not tolerate certain foods at any given time (often dairy or eggs). As the body comes into better balance, some people can relieve their sensitivities.

TREATS

I love chocolate, and I make a raw chocolate pie (from the *Rawfreshing Cuisine* cookbook), as well as many other raw desserts using dates or raw honey as a sweetener. (Beware the evil agave syrup, or raw agave syrup, which is neither raw nor good for you. It reacts with the body the same way high-fructose corn syrup does—adversely.) I make raw brownies frequently and raw cookie dough. I'm also a fan of popcorn popped in coconut oil (always organic) when I need a treat. Raw whipped cream on berries in the summer is hard to beat.

VEGETABLES AND FRUITS

I'm not a big veggie eater. As a yoga teacher, people always think I'm joking when I say that, but the truth is, I dislike chewing through a huge plate of vegetables, and though they are filling, I am not energized enough to complete my daily tasks and I get hungry again within an hour. I love green vegetable drinks because I get a ton of veggies that way, far more than I could ever chew all at once. Using a low-temperature juicer keeps all the live enzymes intact. I'm also a huge fan of microgreens, which are tiny little versions of the big vegetable and carry a huge amount of nutrients in their tiny leaves, actually more than the full-grown vegetable.

I love berries and, like microgreens, they carry huge amounts of benefits despite their little size. Eating too much fruit can get your blood sugar out of balance (which causes an energy "high" followed by a crash and fatigue). Eating raw fats with fruit keeps your energy more balanced. Try cheese and an apple—or my favorite, a bowl of fresh huckleberries covered in raw cacao-cardamom-honey-whipped cream. Yum!

Although it might seem odd to have a nutrition section in a book on yoga, it is important for your overall health that you start to look at yoga with a wider lens. Bring your entire life into a unified whole with the realization that everything affects everything else. Your food carries a vibration, your mind as you're eating carries a vibration, and your digestion is a long process that can be affected at any time and can be the root cause of many diseases if it's not attended to properly. The medicine of Energy Medicine Yoga is the understanding of how much of your life is actually medicine, how you treat and care for your body, with things such as abhyanga and nasya, as well as how and what you eat. This isn't auxiliary to yoga; this *is* yoga. This is the yoga of your life. It takes place off the mat as much as the practices you do on the mat.

11

The Power and Magic of EMYoga: True Transformation

Accept yourself absolutely and unconditionally. It's one of the most radical acts you can do in an insane culture that actually profits from your self-loathing.

TOSHA SILVER

Outrageous Openness: Letting the Divine Take the Lead

How we truly feel about ourselves must be considered when we talk about healing. This chapter is all about the fruition of the EMYoga practice, which leads us to a place of deep intimacy, respect, and love for ourselves. From that place of love and acceptance, change can flow. But first is the place of being with what is. Many of us have what Pema Chödrön calls a "subtle aggression" against ourselves. Unfortunately, our desire for change or transformation often comes from there. But that never works. Transformation begins on its own from deep inside us, when we love ourselves now, just as we are. This is the magic of EMYoga. The way out is in. This may seem paradoxical, that in order to change, we have to accept what is. This is another example of both-and. We *can* change, but first we must accept what is, embrace what is, and allow ourselves to be okay in this moment now.

Part of being able to love yourself is being able to forgive yourself. It is one of the hardest parts of self-reflection—to see yourself truly, to see the things you've done or the times that you have acted less than stellar, less than kind, the times when you've been brusque, dismissive, or worse, cruel to others or yourself.

Often, if you do realize it, you'll beat yourself up for being a bad person. Instead, you must turn to the place of forgiveness—forgiving yourself for your behaviors, forgiving others for their behaviors. This doesn't mean continuing your bad behaviors. It means seeing them, vowing to stop them, and then forgiving yourself. And it doesn't mean allowing people to continue their bad behavior toward you. Forgiving someone doesn't mean you have to befriend them. It simply means you are releasing your anger toward that behavior so you can be free from the anger. It brings you to a very deep place of compassion and can be a turning point on the road to healing.

How you think about yourself broadcasts an energetic frequency. Your thoughts have frequencies. The frequency of your thoughts entrains the frequency of your body to its level. If you've ever stood in front of a mirror and said to yourself, "I hate my body," "I hate my double chin," "I hate my eye sag," "I hate my tits, my big fat gut, my jiggly thighs," "I hate my knobby knees," you are literally entraining your body to disgust and hatred. This affects you more than I could possibly write about in several volumes!

Healing this deep, inner self-loathing ingrained in so many of us is the only way we're going to be able to truly heal the disconnect and divides within ourselves that cause disease. These divides are reflected in the divides in our world that cause a disease of our culture. The racism, hatred, fear, and lack of respect that we project onto others starts within ourselves. We must go there first to unify what is divided.

When we truly love and accept ourselves just as we are, not only accepting our flaws but accepting our essential selves, we are on the path to healing. We draw back to our original, innocent spirit. That place of pure and trusting love and perfection that exists within each of us. In yoga it is called the *purusha*—the untouchable, unbreakable soul. That place is the wellspring of all healing and transformation, because in that place, we are already whole. From there, disease can cease to exist. Also, from the place of the soul is the understanding that sometimes the body is not going to continue on the journey. Then we are freer to release the body and let the soul free.

BREAST HEALTH

One in four women will get breast cancer in her lifetime. The overwhelming toxic load of chemicals in our environment plays a huge role in this, as breast tissue is extremely susceptible to these toxins. Like the canary in a coal mine, breast tissue is some of the first to be toxified and sickened. Add to that the ubiquitous use of underwire bras that restrict the natural movement of the breast as well as the flow of lymph responsible for cleansing these toxins, and it becomes clear how much risk our breasts are under. Donna Eden always encourages women to take the wires or plastics out of their bras or buy wire-free bras, as they are implicated in breast health issues of all kinds.[1]

FOR BREAST HEALTH

Massage the half-moon under the breast to clear toxins and open the natural downward flow of lymph from the delicate breast tissue. The nipple itself is a neurolymphatic point of the Circulation-Sex meridian that carries energy to the protective sac around the heart. Massage the nipples deeply, pressing all the way back toward the rib cage behind the breast. This is detoxifying for the breast and the heart. Then squeeze your breasts firmly. Many women find this deep massage to be uncomfortable or even painful at first. But the more you work these points, the more the pain—in the form of stuck energy and stuck lymph—starts to loosen and release.

A study published by UC Berkeley and the Lawrence Berkeley National Laboratory says squeezing and massaging the breast tissue can help stop cancer by realigning the cells.[2]

LOWER YOUR CANCER RISKS

Remove all chemicals from your life. Start with your body and skin care products. Use only natural, organic products. Many of these are actually less expensive, especially if you research homemade cleaners and balms. Next, go to house and office cleaning products. Particularly disruptive for hormones and also carcinogenic are air fresheners (like Febreze) and chlorines. Then, go to lawn care.

The chemicals that keep your lawn green and free of weeds also put loads of carcinogens in your direct environment and the larger environment. One way to help stop breast cancer and other types of cancers is to stop poisoning ourselves voluntarily.

Gratitude

To feel magic, to feel in the flow of the universe, supported and inspired, is a place we can get to anytime we want. The easiest way to get there is by feeling gratitude. Studies have finally shown us what we already know inside: we are not grateful because we feel happy; we are happy because we feel grateful. Study after study has shown the overwhelming beneficial effects of feeling grateful on both our mental and physical well-being as well as our relationships and our work.

As a culture of overconsumers, many of us have lost the ability to feel thankful. We take and take and never feel complete. Or on the flip side of that, we don't feel we deserve the good things in life and so deny ourselves even the feeling of gratitude. I still remember reading in Laura Ingalls Wilder's book *Little House on the Prairie* about the year that Christmas wasn't going to happen on the prairie because the family was living on an isolated farm and there was no money. Then a friend of Pa's showed up out of a snowstorm, and he gave each of the children a penny. A penny! They were so grateful and happy and full of joy, spinning and dancing and hugging him and each other. I try to remember that when I feel a sense of lack. That a single penny can transform a day!

The place of manifestation, including healing, comes from cultivating gratitude for every aspect of life. We have so much as a culture, and yet we crave ever more. I always keep a gratitude journal by my meditation cushion. In the morning I write down three things I'm grateful for. Every single day. I find this the most powerful when I'm feeling really low, depressed, or despairing. To dig deep and still find gratitude when nothing seems to be going right in my life can be the very thing that helps turn me around and sets me back on my path. Just thinking about what I'm grateful for makes me feel better.

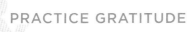

PRACTICE GRATITUDE

In your journal, write down three things a day that you're grateful for. Do this every day for a month.

If you can rewire yourself to feel thankful for what you do have, instead of feeling miserable for what you don't have, you will see the small irritations of your life and the big challenges of your life start to fade. Try spending some time on a regular basis giving thanks for what you already have. Living in a place of gratitude allows big magic in your life. Once you start to welcome in magic—and recognize and give thanks for it—you'll start to see magic show up all over the place. It's like mycelium; its everywhere, just waiting to sprout!

One crucial thing to remember and to feel huge gratitude for on your journey is that you are part of the universe. You are not alone. This is the magic of the Five Elements system. It shows you how every single thing is connected through the matrix of the planetary elements. This is a huge lesson that has been lost due to the limitations of mechanistic science. We are not separate beings alone on a spinning rock, fighting for limited resources. The fact is, we are connected through a unifying field. Call it aether, the Higgs field, the God field—science is still divided on the name. But the existence of a field from which everything arises is undisputed. We are connected to each other—and to every other living thing on this planet—through this field.

This gives us not just a metaphor but a realistic paradigm in which to see ourselves as a true community. We are not isolated, alone, and purposeless. Our actions have consequences to the whole. This is why healing our own self is not a selfish act. As we heal, so the planet heals. If we can change ourselves, we can change the world.

It helps us to be able to see ourselves as part of a whole, instead of just as an individual struggling for survival. And taking that truth into the world is what sparks real actions of change. Again, we must use our both-and adage here. We must heal ourselves within, and then we can heal the world without. This is something to feel hugely grateful for. We are not alone. We are all connected. We are all on the same team!

Body Image, Pleasure, and Sexuality
the Truly Tantric Way

In all my years of teaching yoga I would say that 90 percent or more of the women in my classes were unhappy with their bodies in some way. Whether a woman is thin or plump doesn't seem to matter. Most women are unsatisfied and can pick apart in detail all of their flaws. Their relationship with food is often a battle, and the overwhelming desire to be bone-thin has led some to embrace a vegan or raw food lifestyle as both a means and, just as often, a punishment.

How can EMYoga truly serve you wherever you happen to be in your life, whether on a spiritual path or simply seeking health, calm, equanimity, and joy? The first thing to do, if you're unhappy with your body, is the Temporal Tapping exercise on page 34. This is a powerful tool for rewiring the mind toward self-love. Doing the earth practice (page 174) is also a good place to start.

In a *New York Times* op-ed, I read a quote by the late French philosopher Simone Weil that summed up the essence of the EMYoga practice: "Attention is the rarest and purest form of generosity."[3] Out of context of what the author was writing about, I believe that attention to your own body and mind is the most generous and life-changing thing you can do for yourself. That is what EMYoga is all about, this explicit and deep listening, this attention that you give to yourself.

One of the most profound things we can do is to listen. In our current age, which is smitten by our attachment to i-devices, listening is in short supply. We pay less and less attention to each other or ourselves. And yet, it is the thing we crave the most. We post to Facebook, craving the "likes" of people who take the time to pay attention to us. Our obsession with reality TV is our obsession with being seen, heard, paid attention to.

Instead of fighting for your fifteen minutes of fame, I offer you the EMYoga idea of paying attention to yourself. Spend a little bit, or a lot, of time in which you are deeply and profoundly aware of yourself. When you give yourself this level of attention, you start to learn things about yourself. From knowledge comes awareness, and from awareness comes the ability to transform. So much negative, sarcastic joking has been heaped on "navel gazing" in the New Age world. In fact, this act of deeply looking inward and empowering yourself with true awareness is a revolutionary act.

One of my teacher trainees said that the biggest difference she noticed since practicing EMYoga was her relationship with her body. "I've never touched my body in this way before," she said, laughing. In our culture, we are not encouraged to have a deep intimacy with our own body. We can touch ourselves or another in a sexual way or in a platonic way. If we're parents, we touch our children in a loving way. But we rarely touch ourselves. Let alone daily palpate our bodies to see what they have to report. I've had people in my classes clearing the gates on their feet literally howling with pain, "I've never pressed my feet like this. I had no idea how painful it was!" It was only painful because they didn't touch them. The energies going down to the feet were trapped there and left for dead.

Nothing in your body should hurt. If it does, that is your body trying to send you a signal. Once you start to massage your body, all over your body, and all parts of your body, you begin to see and experience yourself as a whole being. Everything has a story to tell, and everything contains information. Your job is to gather and process that information so you stay healthy. This is a daily practice.

I have a long-haired dog, and every time we come back from a walk in the woods, I check his whole body for burrs and bugs before I let him back in the house. We need to do the same thing to ourselves. A daily check-in to make sure we don't have any "burrs or bugs." This is not only healing and empowering—it feels good.

Part of my mission as a teacher is not only to empower people—to encourage people to think and work outside the box, to reach for their highest potential and become their authentic selves—but to reclaim pleasure.

Imagine if you felt complete, just as you are now. Seriously. Take a moment, close your eyes, and imagine what that would feel like. If there was nothing you desired, nothing you wanted or needed. Everything perfect, just as it is. In our world of constant questing, seeking, building, achieving, consuming, consuming, consuming, it's hard to even imagine that. We are often driven by the things we don't have instead of feeling gratitude for the things we do.

One of the easiest ways I've found to bring pleasure into my life is to cultivate it in my EMYoga practice. Pleasure is something that can exist in almost everything we do. I don't simply mean the pleasure of spending time with friends, or enjoying a good movie, or watching a beautiful sunset, though all of those are extremely important. I mean the visceral, physical pleasure of moving energy in the human body.

According to tantric philosophy, nothing is denied on the path of yoga—this is why tantra is often equated with sex, because sex is not denied as being on the path to enlightenment. The easiest entry into the energetic path of ascending consciousness is through the root chakra. This is also the seat of sexuality, containing, as it does, most of the sexual organs. Mula bandha, the root lock, is located in the first chakra. Prolonged practice with this bandha is known to increase sexual function, performance, and pleasure in both men and women. Most people take the study of tantra no further. But mula bandha is just the starting point to access and illuminate the other chakras, and to access the feeling state of joy, pleasure, and oneness in the physical body and then in the spiritual body. One of the purposes of yoga is to increase upward-moving energy, or *udana*, toward the crown chakra and our connection to the divine—the ultimate feeling of Oneness.

Part of the intrinsically designed beauty of the human body is that our access to God, as it were, is a pleasurable path. It is sensuously pleasurable to move the body, stretch, and open up space for energy. Not only sensual, the feelings in the body as you practice yoga can also feel sexual. This can bring up feelings of denial or shame because of the weighted topic of sexuality in our culture. Many of the role models we've had in our lives for how to be sexual beings are not positive, in part because they never had positive sexual role models. So we have all these mixed signals for how to be sexual beings in the world. There is the oversexualized, the repressed, the exhibitionist, the titillater, but very rarely do we get an appropriate view on a powerful and self-empowered way to own our sexuality.

In a culture of titillating sexuality, we must reclaim what is sacred: the life-force energy itself. That is, in fact, what sexual energy is. It is your life force. And it is no mistake that your life force, flowing through your body, literally *powering* your body through all of its activities, feels good.

This goes back to the beginning of this book and skiers who find powder skiing orgasmic. Unfortunately, we don't have a better language to talk about pleasure, so we sexualize it. The truth is, the body was created in a way that feeling pleasure is its default mode. There is so much of the physical yoga practice that is viscerally pleasurable in that same way. Pleasure is not resigned to the root chakra. You can have an "orgasm" in any of your chakras, meaning, you can feel intense sexual and sensual pleasure in any part of your body. That is the secret behind "more pleasure equals more power."

If we were aware of how easy it is to feel pleasure, and if we accepted that it is not only okay to feel pleasure but that this pleasure can come from doing physical exercise that makes the body healthy, aligns the energy, and promotes healing, we wouldn't be paying millions of dollars to a "health care" industry predicated on the premise that we don't know how to be happy or healthy.

If you can allow yourself the "safe space" to feel pleasure, without inhibition or shame, you are well on your way to reclaiming your own personal power and to being able to create the positive, and sex-positive, life you want. If you have feelings of shame or embarrassment about sex or the physical body, you can use the tapping practices (page 34) to help change those into feelings of empowerment and self-worth.

Your body is a gift and supports everything you do in your life. If you're in a health crisis as you're reading this, you can appreciate even more how a healthy body, no matter the size or shape, is something to prize and treasure. If you are suffering from an injury or an illness, you can still focus on aspects of your body that are working well, even as you try to find solutions to bringing those unwell parts back into balance. Many people use health crises as opportunities to learn and grow, to change bad habits into good ones, and to meditate on a deep appreciation for the positive things in life. I don't want to in any way diminish the challenges of health crises. There are few things worse than being sick or incapacitated to make you feel miserable. But these challenges also offer us insight into how we've previously viewed ourselves.

Hopefully, as you tune and balance your body's energies, you will come more into alignment with a healthy self-image. Throw out the glossy magazines. Look at the celebrity yogi Instagram and Facebook feeds, but make sure you look at a lot of different ones. Look at the skinny yogi and the fleshy yogi, the tall yogi and the short one, men and women of all colors and races and sizes and shapes, and get inspired by the beauty and diversity around you, of which you are a part. Then revel in the strength and individuality of your own body. Affirm all the positive things your body does for you. And tap it in, literally.

R TAP IN JOY

Tap your third eye, between your eyebrows, gently, when you feel joyful, empowered, strong, and happy. It will help imprint that memory in your energy fields.

Embrace your glorious, unique, beautiful self. Then take all that you've learned and share it with someone else. Sister by sister, brother by brother, energy by energy, we can create a healthier, happier world.

Your Own Magic

The most fun I have, bar none, is dropping down into West Bowl on a powder day. The terrain is steep, and when I get fresh tracks, skiing a line that no one has skied yet, I'm giddy and full of joy. Every single cell of my being is engaged in this. There is no part of me that is not joining together in this focused, purposeful movement.

The biggest tip you get once you start skiing off trail in the woods is this: "Look for the white spaces; don't look at the trees. Where you look is where you go." And this, like many skiing metaphors, is a way forward through the challenges of life. Look for the openings; look for the space in between the difficulties. Look for the open doors.

Although the deep snow seems to carry me, I'm working hard to keep everything in balance and on top of a forever-moving target so I can keep it all together. The feeling of joy this brings happens when everything is working in harmony. It happens when I do the work of keeping my body and mind healthy with every tool I have. Then I forget about all the work, and I ski. And it feels like magic.

At the end of the day we're all looking for magic. This includes the ability to affect change, sometimes miraculous change, in our lives at will. EMYoga gives you the path in—a path that is grounded in the physical to help you access both the mental and the spiritual.

It starts at the very physical level of your body. You don't have to remember every point written here. You just have to spend time with your practice. Develop an intimacy with your body. Start to love yourself. Start to feel your energy moving, clearing. Come back daily to the dense physical, and it quickly moves to the more subtle layers. Use the density as a tool to discover where the work needs to be. For a long while, when you're just starting, the work is in the body. First move and release all the energy that is stuck or painful. Get the energy moving again. Your ability to practice this on yourself is the reclamation of your own power. Soon enough, the work starts opening up the channels of mind and spirit. Energy wants to move and flow, and once you start to listen to it and tune in, it will take you on amazing journeys.

The healing journey I take most often is to walk barefoot. Any time I can, I plug myself into the earth's energy to help bring my body back to a neutral, calm, and energized place. I tell everyone to plug themselves in, to access the free, abundant, healing energy of the planet. In fact, the best way to practice EMYoga is directly on the earth. This is my preferred way to practice, gathering in the planet's energy and hooking my own energy in with it at the same time. I love to press my face into the fresh grass as I'm lying on my belly. I love to have my hands and feet pressed into the dirt or the sand or the grass. Use a yoga blanket to help align your practice or add padding, but let yourself touch bare earth as much as you can. And don't just take your shoes off. Take off your outside layer, your house or your car or your jacket. Take off your civilization and get out into the natural world. Go somewhere quiet, where there is only water or wind in the trees or bugs clacking. Get to a place beyond buzzing and motors and Wi-Fi and interceptions. If you can, do this once a week—at the very least. If you're compelled to do more, then by all means the more you immerse yourself in the natural world, hiking for a full day, camping out spending 24 or 76 or 108 hours with the bugs and all, the better you will feel. It is a powerful healer. And when you merge back into your life, it will remain with you. The silence between the beats. You can find pockets of nature even in a bustling city. Stop near a tree and place your hands on its bark. Breathe in its fresh air. Even this small amount of stop in your day is powerfully healing.

The trick to living this life is to stay with yourself. So often, we leave. We run or obscure or deny or hide from ourselves in a million ways. The power of EMYoga is that it helps show you a way to come back to yourself and to stay with yourself. A health crisis, an emotional crisis, or a spiritual crisis are all times we can check out. But we tend to check out no matter what is going on. We're always on our phones, computers, TVs. We don't schedule relaxation time, time to do nothing and simply be still. We need to learn and practice staying present and being still, receptive, open.

When your body or mind goes into fear or anger, or an illness descends, you need to learn to treat yourself with compassion as if you were a small child again. Only now, you will do the ministering, the mothering, and the fathering to yourself, instead of looking to the outside world to help you. This is the start of self-love and self-compassion, and it is the place you need to get to in order to feel whole and at ease. No one but you knows exactly how it is inside your specific being. No one but you knows exactly what you need to salve your wounds.

Many of the practices in EMYoga are about holds—holding the head, holding the body in a hug, holding points, holding and rocking. This is more than simply the metaphor of "holding onto yourself"—these practices elicit healing responses from the energetics of the body.

When I'm going through something difficult, I notice my own tendencies to want to run away and hide. This is how my water expresses itself when I'm out of balance. And when I'm going through something difficult, I'm frequently out of balance. Beyond all the holds and practices here, I'll often start with something very, very simple. I'll sit or lie down and hold one or both hands over my heart. I'll first start to just listen to my heartbeat. That is the initial way in. If things are really bad, it might take a long time for me to feel it. After a time, the heartbeat will become strong, and I'll start to feel a softening and an opening. Almost as if my chest itself is opening. Almost as if I could hold my actual heart in my hands. Then I feel my heartbeat on another level. I feel it holding me, surrounding me, and bathing me in the coherent resonance of love and light that is my inherent nature. Bringing me back into the harmony of my own being.

This, at the end of it all, is the deepest power and source of yoga. The light within. The love within. It is there, at all times, waiting to hold you. And when you surrender to it, to yourself, to your own love, you find a resilience that might surprise you.

Your whole life might surprise you.

You just have to let it.

Acknowledgments

Thank You . . . You inspired me from the first moment to be better, stronger, happier, more resilient. To question everything. To search tirelessly for truth. To be courageous and impeccable with my words. I have tried, with every fiber of my being, to be this, and to also be kind.

Thank you to my teachers, Donna Eden and David Feinstein, whose continued presence in my life is a blessing of the highest order. They are the perfect representation of the yin and yang working seamlessly together to produce much more than the sum of the parts. They are changing the way we think about energy and healing, and I am blessed to count them not only as my teachers but also as my friends.

My mother, Rachel Walker, a writer in her own right, continues to support me on my path no matter what twists and turns it takes or how many obstacles arise. Our relationship is complex and challenging and is a continual source of inspiration and strength, and I am so grateful to have a mother who broke the mold with her own life, so I had it a little easier breaking the mold of mine.

My father, a shining angel who continues to inspire me and who I strive to make proud with everything I do.

A huge thank you to my sister, Jennifer, always my first reader, most discerning critic, and biggest ally.

To my whole family, East Coast and West, who support and love me and give me the confidence to pursue my passions.

Thank you to my dear friends and sanity keepers during the writing of this book: Jesse Devine, Mary Person, Stephanie Elm, Ingrid Wick, Jenny Wickland, Ryan Wickland, and Eileen McKusick. Thank you to my bonus family the Koch-Fords: Paula, Matt, Ammann, JP, and Lilly, for always taking care of Louis when I have to travel, and for taking care of me when I'm home. Thank you to Soña Hernandez, for all your help with the book, and for the magic. #tymp

Thank you, Gigi Rappaport and Sue Purvis, for giving me up-to-the-minute ski reports, so I could make a smart decision whether to ski or to work.

Heather Maidat and Sue P., for the professional writing talk that helps so much during the isolated time of writing a book.

Mollie Silver, for being the amazing first pair of eyes to read the practices in this book. You are a true, wise gem.

Elaine Doll, for your Ayurvedic teachings and magnificent friendship. Kathryn Hayes, for your incredible everythingness. You are a metal star!

Sherri Nicholas, for your passion and artistry with EM and EMYoga.

To my whole Innersource family who work tirelessly promoting Donna's work, especially Michelle Earnest, for her valuable contributions to this book, and Roger Devenyns and Jeffrey McDonnell, for keeping it all together. To Innersource teachers Susan Stone, Sara Allen, and Lisa Buford for your help with and powerful contributions to this book. To Cheryl Lee, Katerina Kostova Crews, Kelmie Blake, Deirdre Áine McGrath, and the whole Innersource community, who are always available and inspired for questions, troubleshooting, and support with all things EM.

To Dondi Dahlin for your brilliance and support. Thank you to Titanya Dahlin for setting me on this path. And to both of you for being my amazing EM sisters!

Brett Tallman, for explaining EMFs in a simple way. Dr. Heather Tallman Ruhm, for your contributions to the nutrition section, and for corroborating from an MD perspective so much of what I'm teaching.

Thank you to my whole team at Sounds True who push me to produce my best work, even when I try to resist: Jennifer Brown, Haven Iverson, and the tireless, amazing, patient, and wonderful Gretel Hakanson. Thank you to Brooks Freehill, Rachael Murray, Beth Skelley, and Jen Murphy for a fun and successful photo shoot—despite my 103 degree fever—and for making this book beautiful. Thank you to Haven Collective for the beautiful clothes, MaxandJane.com for the skin care, and Brandi Young for the rad haircut. Thanks to Stephen Lessard, Hayden Peltier, Drummond West, Samantha Erickson, Aron Arnold, and Solay Howell for helping realize my vision for the video shoot and for making it seamless and a perfect companion to the book. To Dee Sandella, for the perfect hair and makeup. Jade Lascelles and Jody Berman, for their conscientious up leveling of this book, I am forever grateful.

Susan Nichols, Steve Garretson, and Kim Collier for their unwavering support and honest companies. Craig Weiner and Alina Frank for your support and clarity.

To the amazing, groundbreaking, and mind-expanding scientists who continue to challenge me and break down dogma: Dr. James L. Oschman, Dr. Rupert Sheldrake, Dr. Candace B. Pert, and Dr. Bruce H. Lipton. Thank you to Merlin and Cosmo Sheldrake, who along with Rupert, helped inspire me to bring magic into my work with the magic they bring to theirs.

Dr. John Douillard, for your unending wisdom and generosity in sharing your knowledge with as many people as possible.

Thank you to all my yoga teachers who have fed me when I was hungry and helped to bring light into the darkness. Especially to Ram Dass, who gave me my first glimpse into the yoga world with your supercool book, *Be Here Now*, which I read as a child, and for being so full of wisdom and compassion when I finally got the chance to sit with you as an adult.

Thank you to all my EMYoga teachers, who passionately take up these books and bring this work out into the world. And to all my students, who teach me more than you could ever possibly know.

∞

This book is lovingly dedicated to Lorin Kim Walker—my namesake, my favorite uncle, the one who brought me out west for the first time, changing my life forever—who died during the writing of this book.

And to all of those who died too young . . .

Notes

Chapter 1

1. Jenn Bodnar, "Healing vs. Fixing: An Interview with Mathew Sanford," *Yoga Digest*, April 2015, 25.

2. Christiane Northrup, *Goddesses Never Age: The Secret Prescription for Radiance, Vitality, and Well-Being* (Carlsbad, CA: Hay House, 2015), 9.

3. Joe Dispenza, *You Are the Placebo: Making Your Mind Matter* (Carlsbad, CA: Hay House, 2015).

4. Deepak Chopra, *Perfect Health: The Complete Mind/Body Guide* (New York: Three Rivers Press, 2000), 17.

5. Norman Doidge, *The Brain's Way of Healing: Remarkable Discoveries and Recoveries from the Frontiers of Neuroplasticity* (New York: Penguin Books, 2015), 31.

6. Bruce H. Lipton, *The Biology of Belief : Unleashing the Power of Consciousness, Matter, & Miracles* (Fulton, CA: Elite Books, 2005).

7. James L. Oschman, *Energy Medicine: The Scientific Basis* (London: Churchill Livingstone, 2000), 232.

8. Rupert Sheldrake, *The Presence of Past: Morphic Resonance and the Memory of Nature* (South Paris, ME: Park Street Press, 2012).

9. Andrew Weil, *Spontaneous Healing: How to Discover and Embrace Your Body's Natural Ability to Maintain and Heal Itself* (New York: Ballantine Books, 2000), 92.

10. National Cancer Institute, Surveillance, Epidemiology, and End Results Program, "SEER Stat Fact Sheets: Cancer of Any Site," seer.cancer.gov/statfacts/html/all.html.

11. S. D. Wells, "75% of Physicians in the World Refuse Chemotherapy for Themselves," *Natural News*, January 13, 2012, naturalnews.com/036054_chemotherapy_physicians_toxicity.html.

12. The ECS Therapy Center, myecstherapy.org.

13. Mercola.com, "A New View of Cancer—German New Medicine," September 8, 2007, articles.mercola.com/sites/articles/archive/2007/09/08 /a-new-view-of-cancer-german-new-medicine.aspx.

Chapter 2

1. John Douillard, "Episode 10: Love, Sex and Yoga," podcast, June 9, 2014, lifespa.com/webinar-love-sex-yoga.

2. Angie LeVan, "Seeing Is Believing: The Power of Visualization," *Psychology Today*, December 3, 2009, psychologytoday.com/blog/flourish/200912 /seeing-is-believing-the-power-visualization.

3. Donna Eden with David Feinstein, *Energy Medicine: Balancing Your Body's Energies for Optimal Health, Joy, and Vitality* (New York: Jeremy P. Tarcher, 2008).

Chapter 3

1. Dondi Dahlin, *The Five Elements: Understand Yourself and Enhance Your Relationships with the Wisdom of the World's Oldest Personality Type System* (New York: TarcherPerigree, 2016), 7.

2. Donna Eden, "Eden Energy Medicine Certification Program," Innersource class handout, 13.

3. Candace B. Pert, *Molecules of Emotion: The Science Behind Mind-Body Medicine* (New York: Touchstone, 1997).

4. Ibid., 192.

5. Harriet Beinfield and Efrem Korngold, *Between Heaven and Earth: A Guide to Chinese Medicine* (New York: Ballantine, 1991), 45.

6. Ibid., 87.

7. Bruce Lipton, "Evolution by BITs and Pieces: An Introduction to Fractal Evolution," June 7, 2012, brucelipton.com/resource/article/fractal-evolution.

Chapter 4

1. Oschman, *Energy Medicine*, 252.

Chapter 6

1. Marianne Williamson, *A Return to Love: Reflections on the Principles of A Course in Miracles* (New York: HarperCollins, 1992), 190–91.

2. Agnes De Mille, *Martha: The Life and Work of Martha Graham—A Biography* (New York: Random House, 1991).

Chapter 8

1. Sara Allen, "Earth Energy Heals Everything," Innersource class handout, 2015, 10.

2. Ibid., 11.

3. Ibid., 16.

4. Ibid., 11.

5. Choa Kok Sui, *SuperBrain Yoga* (Quezon City, Philippines: Institute for Inner Studies Publishing Foundation, Inc., 2005).

6. John Douillard, *Body, Mind, & Sport: The Mind-Body Guide to Lifelong Health, Fitness, and Your Personal Best*, rev. ed. (New York: Three Rivers Press, 2001), 143.

7. Donna Eden with David Feinstein, *Energy Medicine for Women: Aligning Your Body's Energies to Boost Your Health and Vitality* (New York: TarcherPerigree, 2008), 124.

8. Ibid., 116.

9. Douillard, *Body, Mind, & Sport*, 146.

10. Ibid., 146.

Chapter 9

1. "Grief and Praise Part 1," YouTube video, 21:36, from a talk by Martin Prechtel, posted by the Emowell Project, February 19, 2014, youtube.com /watch?v=h6h3JNOCTYc.

Chapter 10

1. Joseph Mercola, "Why Smells Can Trigger Strong Memories," August 6, 2015, articles.mercola.com/sites/articles/archive/2015/08/06/smells-trigger-memories.aspx.

2. "Nasal Cleansing with Nasya," September 17, 2010, flowingfree.org /ayurvedic-remedy-nasal-cleansing-with-nasya.

3. Weil, *Spontaneous Healing*.

4. *Microwave News*, "Cell Phone Radiation Boosts Cancer Rates in Animals; $25 Million NTP Study Finds Brain Tumors," microwavenews.com /news-center/ntp-cancer-results.

5. Author's personal conversation with Brett Tallman, spring 2016.

6. Rob Knight and Brendan Buhler, *Follow Your Gut: The Enormous Impact of Tiny Microbes* (New York: Simon & Schuster, 2015).

7. Sarah Yang, "To Revert Breast Cancer Cells, Give Them the Squeeze," *Berkeley News*, December 17, 2012, news.berkeley.edu/2012/12/17 /malignant-breast-cells-grow-normally-when-compressed.

8. Aajonus Vonderplanitz, *We Want to Live* (Los Angeles: Carnelian Bay Castle Press, 1997), 146–47.

9. Ibid., 147.

10. T. K. V. Desikachar, *The Heart of Yoga: Developing a Personal Practice* (Rochester, VT: Inner Traditions, 1995), 98.

11. Medical Medium's Facebook page, November 16, 2016, facebook.com /medicalmedium/posts/900659513402561.

12. Sally Fallon and Mary G. Enig, *Nourishing Traditions: The Cookbook that Challenges Politically Correct Nutrition and the Diet Dictocrats* (Washington, DC: New Trends, 1999), 610.

Chapter 11

1. Mercola.com, "Can Wearing Your Bra Cause Cancer?" May 19, 2009,
    articles.mercola.com/sites/articles/archive/2009/05/19/Can-Wearing-Your
    -Bra-Cause-Cancer.aspx#_edn2; Habib Sadeghi, "Could There Possibly Be
    a Link Between Underwire Bras and Breast Cancer??," *Goop*, goop.com
    /could-there-possibly-be-a-link-between-underwire-bras-and-breast-cancer/.

2. Yang, "To Revert Breast Cancer Cells, Give Them the Squeeze."

3. Jonathan Safran Foer, "How Not to Be Alone," *New York Times*, June 8, 2013,
    nytimes.com/2013/06/09/opinion/sunday/how-not-to-be-alone.html.

Resources

Energy Medicine

Energy Medicine: Balancing Your Body's Energies for Optimal Health, Joy, and Vitality
   by Donna Eden with David Feinstein

*Energy Medicine for Women: Aligning Your Body's Energies to Boost Your Health
   and Vitality* by Donna Eden with David Feinstein

*The Promise of Energy Medicine Psychology: Revolutionary Tools for Dramatic Personal
   Change* by David Feinstein, Donna Eden, and Gary Craig

To become a certified EM practitioner, or to find a certified EM practitioner,
   go to Innersource.net.

EMYoga

To become a certified EMYoga teacher, go to EMYoga.net.

For many of the products and books that I use and recommend,
   go to EMYoga.net/resources.

Ayurvedic Research, Classes, Information, Supplements, and Products

John Douillard's LifeSpa: LifeSpa.com

Elaine Doll's Blissful Ayurveda: blissfulbozeman.com

Emotional Freedom Technique Tapping

EFT Tapping Training: efttappingtraining.com

Home for Official EFT: emofree.com

Cancer and Illness Resources

The ECS Therapy Center: myecstherapy.org

The Germanic New Medicine: newmedicine.ca

Hippocrites Health Institute: hippocratesinst.org

The Truth About Cancer: thetruthaboutcancer.com

Health Resources

Integrative physician Heather Tallman Ruhm, MD: drtallmanruhm.com

Julie Schleusner, DC: bigskywellnesscenter.com, 406.755.4119

Other Resources

Bruce H. Lipton: brucelipton.com

Fractals movie, *Zero Point: Volume II—The Structure of Infinity*:
  youtube.com/watch?v=S2rg7CeY1ek

You Are the Placebo: Making the Mind Matter by Joe Dispenza

Index

Page numbers in italics refer to figures; **page numbers in bold refer to tables.**

Practice sequences are noted in parentheses.

About the Author

Lauren Walker has been teaching yoga and meditation since 1997. She splits her time between New England and Montana. A writer since childhood, Lauren publishes widely and has written features for the *New York Times*, the *Jerusalem Post*, and Salon.com. She has been featured in *Yoga Journal, Mantra Yoga + Health*, and *Yoga Digest*, and was named one of the top one hundred most influential yoga teachers in the United States. Lauren is a wandering spirit and has lived and worked all over the world. She continues to travel and teach in the United States, Canada, and abroad. Lauren is also a composer, diehard skier, outdoorswoman, and passionate advocate for a healthy planet. For more on Lauren and Energy Medicine Yoga, please visit EMYoga.net.

About Sounds True

Sounds True is a multimedia publisher whose mission is to inspire and support personal transformation and spiritual awakening. Founded in 1985 and located in Boulder, Colorado, we work with many of the leading spiritual teachers, thinkers, healers, and visionary artists of our time. We strive with every title to preserve the essential "living wisdom" of the author or artist. It is our goal to create products that not only provide information to a reader or listener, but that also embody the quality of a wisdom transmission.

For those seeking genuine transformation, Sounds True is your trusted partner. At SoundsTrue.com you will find a wealth of free resources to support your journey, including exclusive weekly audio interviews, free downloads, interactive learning tools, and other special savings on all our titles.

To learn more, please visit SoundsTrue.com/freegifts or call us toll-free at 800.333.9185.

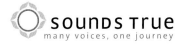

SOUNDS TRUE
many voices, one journey